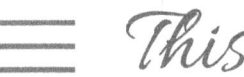

CAREGIVER BOOK
Belongs to:

NAME : _____

PHONE : _____

EMAIL : _____

ADDRESS : _____

_____

EMERGENCY CONTACT LIST

EMERGENCY CONTACTS

CONTACT 1 NAME		RELATIONSHIP	
PHONE 1		PHONE 2	
ADDRESS			
CONTACT 2 NAME		RELATIONSHIP	
PHONE 1		PHONE 2	
ADDRESS			
CONTACT 3 NAME		RELATIONSHIP	
PHONE 1		PHONE 2	
ADDRESS			

NEIGHBORS / LANDLORD / HOA

NEIGHBOR 1 NAME		PHONE	
NEIGHBOR 2 NAME		PHONE	
NEIGHBOR 3 NAME		PHONE	
LANDLORD / HOA		PHONE	

MEDICAL CONTACT INFO

DOCTOR NAME		PHONE	
DENTIST NAME		PHONE	
PREFERRED HOSPITAL		PHONE	

POLICE / AMBULANCE / FIRE :

POLICE DEPARTMENT		PHONE	
FIRE DEPARTMENT		PHONE	
ELECTRIC COMPANY		PHONE	
GAS COMPANY		PHONE	
WATER COMPANY		PHONE	
POISON CONTROL		PHONE	
ANIMAL CONTROL		PHONE	

DATE:

TOILET / DIAPER

TIME	RESULT	
:	wet	b.m.
:	wet	b.m.
:	wet	b.m.
:	wet	b.m.
:	wet	b.m.
:	wet	b.m.
:	wet	b.m.

MEALS / FEEDINGS

TIME	AMOUNT
:	
:	
:	
:	
:	
:	
:	

PERSONAL CARE

☐ Shower ☐ Bed Bath ☐ Brush Hair ☐ Teeth

PHYSICAL THERAPY

☐ Back ☐ Neck ☐ Shoulders
☐ Arms ☐ Hands ☐ Legs ☐ Feet
☐ Speech Therapy

SPECIAL CARE

MEDICINE	DOSAGE	TIME	MEDICINE	DOSAGE	TIME
		:			:
		:			:
		:			:
		:			:
		:			:
		:			:

BLOOD PRESSURE

SYSTOLIC	DIASTOLIC	TIME
		:
		:
		:
		:
		:
		:

ACTIVITIES

ACTIVITY	LENGTH

SUPPLIES NEEDED

NOTES

LEVEL OF HAPPINESS AM: ☐☐☐☐ PM: ☐☐☐☐
NOTES: _____
_____

LEVEL OF ENGAGEMENT AM: ☐☐☐☐ PM: ☐☐☐☐
NOTES: _____
_____

LEVEL OF DISCOMFORT AM: ☐☐☐☐ PM: ☐☐☐☐
NOTES: _____
_____

LEVEL OF SLEEP AM: ☐☐☐☐ PM: ☐☐☐☐
NOTES: _____
_____

Are you noticing anything different today?
_____
_____

What is your ongoing or new goal for success in caregiving and helping your loved one to age gracefully and in a way that first their individual need and disposition?
_____
_____
_____

What were your challenges and triumphs today?
_____
_____

Do you have any questions or concerns to reach out about?
_____
_____

DATE:

TOILET / DIAPER

TIME	RESULT	
:	wet	b.m.
:	wet	b.m.
:	wet	b.m.
:	wet	b.m.
:	wet	b.m.
:	wet	b.m.
:	wet	b.m.

MEALS / FEEDINGS

TIME	AMOUNT
:	
:	
:	
:	
:	
:	
:	

PERSONAL CARE

☐ Shower ☐ Bed Bath ☐ Brush Hair ☐ Teeth

PHYSICAL THERAPY

☐ Back ☐ Neck ☐ Shoulders
☐ Arms ☐ Hands ☐ Legs ☐ Feet
☐ Speech Therapy

SPECIAL CARE

MEDICINE	DOSAGE	TIME	MEDICINE	DOSAGE	TIME
		:			:
		:			:
		:			:
		:			:
		:			:
		:			:

BLOOD PRESSURE

SYSTOLIC	DIASTOLIC	TIME
		:
		:
		:
		:
		:
		:

ACTIVITIES

ACTIVITY	LENGTH

SUPPLIES NEEDED

NOTES

LEVEL OF HAPPINESS　　AM: ☐☐☐☐☐　　PM: ☐☐☐☐☐

NOTES: _____

_____

LEVEL OF ENGAGEMENT　AM: ☐☐☐☐☐　　PM: ☐☐☐☐☐

NOTES: _____

_____

LEVEL OF DISCOMFORT　AM: ☐☐☐☐☐　　PM: ☐☐☐☐☐

NOTES: _____

_____

LEVEL OF SLEEP　　　　AM: ☐☐☐☐☐　　PM: ☐☐☐☐☐

NOTES: _____

_____

Are you noticing anything different today?

_____

_____

What is your ongoing or new goal for success in caregiving and helping your loved one to age gracefully and in a way that first their individual need and disposition?

_____

_____

_____

What were your challenges and triumphs today?

_____

_____

Do you have any questions or concerns to reach out about?

_____

_____

DATE:

TOILET / DIAPER

TIME	RESULT	
:	wet	b.m.
:	wet	b.m.
:	wet	b.m.
:	wet	b.m.
:	wet	b.m.
:	wet	b.m.
:	wet	b.m.

MEALS / FEEDINGS

TIME	AMOUNT
:	
:	
:	
:	
:	
:	
:	

PERSONAL CARE

☐ Shower ☐ Bed Bath ☐ Brush Hair ☐ Teeth

PHYSICAL THERAPY

☐ Back ☐ Neck ☐ Shoulders
☐ Arms ☐ Hands ☐ Legs ☐ Feet
☐ Speech Therapy

SPECIAL CARE

MEDICINE	DOSAGE	TIME	MEDICINE	DOSAGE	TIME
		:			:
		:			:
		:			:
		:			:
		:			:
		:			:

BLOOD PRESSURE

SYSTOLIC	DIASTOLIC	TIME
		:
		:
		:
		:
		:
		:

ACTIVITIES

ACTIVITY	LENGTH

SUPPLIES NEEDED

NOTES

LEVEL OF HAPPINESS AM: ☐☐☐☐☐ PM: ☐☐☐☐☐
NOTES: _____
_____

LEVEL OF ENGAGEMENT AM: ☐☐☐☐☐ PM: ☐☐☐☐☐
NOTES: _____
_____

LEVEL OF DISCOMFORT AM: ☐☐☐☐☐ PM: ☐☐☐☐☐
NOTES: _____
_____

LEVEL OF SLEEP AM: ☐☐☐☐☐ PM: ☐☐☐☐☐
NOTES: _____
_____

Are you noticing anything different today?
_____
_____

What is your ongoing or new goal for success in caregiving and helping your loved one to age gracefully and in a way that first their individual need and disposition?
_____
_____
_____

What were your challenges and triumphs today?
_____
_____

Do you have any questions or concerns to reach out about?
_____
_____

DATE:

TOILET / DIAPER

TIME	RESULT	
:	wet	b.m.
:	wet	b.m.
:	wet	b.m.
:	wet	b.m.
:	wet	b.m.
:	wet	b.m.
:	wet	b.m.

MEALS / FEEDINGS

TIME	AMOUNT
:	
:	
:	
:	
:	
:	
:	

PERSONAL CARE

☐ Shower ☐ Bed Bath ☐ Brush Hair ☐ Teeth

PHYSICAL THERAPY

☐ Back ☐ Neck ☐ Shoulders
☐ Arms ☐ Hands ☐ Legs ☐ Feet
☐ Speech Therapy

SPECIAL CARE

MEDICINE	DOSAGE	TIME	MEDICINE	DOSAGE	TIME
		:			:
		:			:
		:			:
		:			:
		:			:
		:			:

BLOOD PRESSURE

SYSTOLIC	DIASTOLIC	TIME
		:
		:
		:
		:
		:
		:

ACTIVITIES

ACTIVITY	LENGTH

SUPPLIES NEEDED

NOTES

LEVEL OF HAPPINESS   AM: ☐☐☐☐☐   PM: ☐☐☐☐☐

NOTES: _____

_____

LEVEL OF ENGAGEMENT   AM: ☐☐☐☐☐   PM: ☐☐☐☐☐

NOTES: _____

_____

LEVEL OF DISCOMFORT   AM: ☐☐☐☐☐   PM: ☐☐☐☐☐

NOTES: _____

_____

LEVEL OF SLEEP   AM: ☐☐☐☐☐   PM: ☐☐☐☐☐

NOTES: _____

_____

Are you noticing anything different today?

_____

_____

What is your ongoing or new goal for success in caregiving and helping your loved one to age gracefully and in a way that first their individual need and disposition?

_____

_____

_____

What were your challenges and triumphs today?

_____

_____

Do you have any questions or concerns to reach out about?

_____

_____

DATE:

TOILET / DIAPER

TIME	RESULT	
:	wet	b.m.
:	wet	b.m.
:	wet	b.m.
:	wet	b.m.
:	wet	b.m.
:	wet	b.m.
:	wet	b.m.

MEALS / FEEDINGS

TIME	AMOUNT
:	
:	
:	
:	
:	
:	
:	

PERSONAL CARE

☐ Shower ☐ Bed Bath ☐ Brush Hair ☐ Teeth

PHYSICAL THERAPY

☐ Back ☐ Neck ☐ Shoulders
☐ Arms ☐ Hands ☐ Legs ☐ Feet
☐ Speech Therapy

SPECIAL CARE

MEDICINE	DOSAGE	TIME	MEDICINE	DOSAGE	TIME
		:			:
		:			:
		:			:
		:			:
		:			:
		:			:

BLOOD PRESSURE

SYSTOLIC	DIASTOLIC	TIME
		:
		:
		:
		:
		:
		:

ACTIVITIES

ACTIVITY	LENGTH

SUPPLIES NEEDED

NOTES

LEVEL OF HAPPINESS   AM: ☐☐☐☐☐   PM: ☐☐☐☐☐
NOTES: _____
_____

LEVEL OF ENGAGEMENT   AM: ☐☐☐☐☐   PM: ☐☐☐☐☐
NOTES: _____
_____

LEVEL OF DISCOMFORT   AM: ☐☐☐☐☐   PM: ☐☐☐☐☐
NOTES: _____
_____

LEVEL OF SLEEP   AM: ☐☐☐☐☐   PM: ☐☐☐☐☐
NOTES: _____
_____

Are you noticing anything different today?
_____
_____

What is your ongoing or new goal for success in caregiving and helping your loved one to age gracefully and in a way that first their individual need and disposition?
_____
_____
_____

What were your challenges and triumphs today?
_____
_____

Do you have any questions or concerns to reach out about?
_____
_____

DATE:

TOILET / DIAPER

TIME	RESULT	
:	wet	b.m.
:	wet	b.m.
:	wet	b.m.
:	wet	b.m.
:	wet	b.m.
:	wet	b.m.
:	wet	b.m.

MEALS / FEEDINGS

TIME	AMOUNT
:	
:	
:	
:	
:	
:	
:	

PERSONAL CARE

☐ Shower ☐ Bed Bath ☐ Brush Hair ☐ Teeth

PHYSICAL THERAPY

☐ Back ☐ Neck ☐ Shoulders
☐ Arms ☐ Hands ☐ Legs ☐ Feet
☐ Speech Therapy

SPECIAL CARE

MEDICINE	DOSAGE	TIME	MEDICINE	DOSAGE	TIME
		:			:
		:			:
		:			:
		:			:
		:			:
		:			:

BLOOD PRESSURE

SYSTOLIC	DIASTOLIC	TIME
		:
		:
		:
		:
		:
		:

ACTIVITIES

ACTIVITY	LENGTH

SUPPLIES NEEDED

NOTES

LEVEL OF HAPPINESS   AM: ☐☐☐☐☐   PM: ☐☐☐☐☐
NOTES: _____
_____

LEVEL OF ENGAGEMENT   AM: ☐☐☐☐☐   PM: ☐☐☐☐☐
NOTES: _____
_____

LEVEL OF DISCOMFORT   AM: ☐☐☐☐☐   PM: ☐☐☐☐☐
NOTES: _____
_____

LEVEL OF SLEEP   AM: ☐☐☐☐☐   PM: ☐☐☐☐☐
NOTES: _____
_____

Are you noticing anything different today?
_____
_____

What is your ongoing or new goal for success in caregiving and helping your loved one to age gracefully and in a way that first their individual need and disposition?
_____
_____
_____

What were your challenges and triumphs today?
_____
_____

Do you have any questions or concerns to reach out about?
_____
_____

DATE:

TOILET / DIAPER

TIME	RESULT	
:	wet	b.m.
:	wet	b.m.
:	wet	b.m.
:	wet	b.m.
:	wet	b.m.
:	wet	b.m.
:	wet	b.m.

MEALS / FEEDINGS

TIME	AMOUNT
:	
:	
:	
:	
:	
:	
:	

PERSONAL CARE

☐ Shower ☐ Bed Bath ☐ Brush Hair ☐ Teeth

PHYSICAL THERAPY

☐ Back ☐ Neck ☐ Shoulders
☐ Arms ☐ Hands ☐ Legs ☐ Feet
☐ Speech Therapy

SPECIAL CARE

MEDICINE	DOSAGE	TIME	MEDICINE	DOSAGE	TIME
		:			:
		:			:
		:			:
		:			:
		:			:
		:			:

BLOOD PRESSURE

SYSTOLIC	DIASTOLIC	TIME
		:
		:
		:
		:
		:
		:

ACTIVITIES

ACTIVITY	LENGTH

SUPPLIES NEEDED

NOTES

LEVEL OF HAPPINESS AM: ☐☐☐☐   PM: ☐☐☐☐
NOTES: _____
_____

LEVEL OF ENGAGEMENT AM: ☐☐☐☐   PM: ☐☐☐☐
NOTES: _____
_____

LEVEL OF DISCOMFORT AM: ☐☐☐☐   PM: ☐☐☐☐
NOTES: _____
_____

LEVEL OF SLEEP AM: ☐☐☐☐   PM: ☐☐☐☐
NOTES: _____
_____

Are you noticing anything different today?
_____
_____

What is your ongoing or new goal for success in caregiving and helping your loved one to age gracefully and in a way that first their individual need and disposition?
_____
_____
_____

What were your challenges and triumphs today?
_____
_____

Do you have any questions or concerns to reach out about?
_____
_____

DATE:

TOILET / DIAPER

TIME	RESULT	
:	wet	b.m.
:	wet	b.m.
:	wet	b.m.
:	wet	b.m.
:	wet	b.m.
:	wet	b.m.
:	wet	b.m.

MEALS / FEEDINGS

TIME	AMOUNT
:	
:	
:	
:	
:	
:	
:	

PERSONAL CARE

☐ Shower ☐ Bed Bath ☐ Brush Hair ☐ Teeth

PHYSICAL THERAPY

☐ Back ☐ Neck ☐ Shoulders
☐ Arms ☐ Hands ☐ Legs ☐ Feet
☐ Speech Therapy

SPECIAL CARE

MEDICINE	DOSAGE	TIME	MEDICINE	DOSAGE	TIME
		:			:
		:			:
		:			:
		:			:
		:			:
		:			:

BLOOD PRESSURE

SYSTOLIC	DIASTOLIC	TIME
		:
		:
		:
		:
		:
		:

ACTIVITIES

ACTIVITY	LENGTH

SUPPLIES NEEDED

NOTES

LEVEL OF HAPPINESS AM: [ ][ ][ ][ ][ ]   PM: [ ][ ][ ][ ][ ]
NOTES: _____
_____

LEVEL OF ENGAGEMENT AM: [ ][ ][ ][ ][ ]   PM: [ ][ ][ ][ ][ ]
NOTES: _____
_____

LEVEL OF DISCOMFORT AM: [ ][ ][ ][ ][ ]   PM: [ ][ ][ ][ ][ ]
NOTES: _____
_____

LEVEL OF SLEEP AM: [ ][ ][ ][ ][ ]   PM: [ ][ ][ ][ ][ ]
NOTES: _____
_____

Are you noticing anything different today?
_____
_____

What is your ongoing or new goal for success in caregiving and helping your loved one to age gracefully and in a way that first their individual need and disposition?
_____
_____

What were your challenges and triumphs today?
_____
_____

Do you have any questions or concerns to reach out about?
_____
_____

DATE:

TOILET / DIAPER

TIME	RESULT	
:	wet	b.m.
:	wet	b.m.
:	wet	b.m.
:	wet	b.m.
:	wet	b.m.
:	wet	b.m.
:	wet	b.m.

MEALS / FEEDINGS

TIME	AMOUNT
:	
:	
:	
:	
:	
:	
:	

PERSONAL CARE

☐ Shower ☐ Bed Bath ☐ Brush Hair ☐ Teeth

PHYSICAL THERAPY

☐ Back ☐ Neck ☐ Shoulders
☐ Arms ☐ Hands ☐ Legs ☐ Feet
☐ Speech Therapy

SPECIAL CARE

MEDICINE	DOSAGE	TIME	MEDICINE	DOSAGE	TIME
		:			:
		:			:
		:			:
		:			:
		:			:
		:			:

BLOOD PRESSURE

SYSTOLIC	DIASTOLIC	TIME
		:
		:
		:
		:
		:
		:

ACTIVITIES

ACTIVITY	LENGTH

SUPPLIES NEEDED

NOTES

LEVEL OF HAPPINESS AM: ☐☐☐☐☐   PM: ☐☐☐☐☐
NOTES: _____
_____

LEVEL OF ENGAGEMENT AM: ☐☐☐☐☐   PM: ☐☐☐☐☐
NOTES: _____
_____

LEVEL OF DISCOMFORT AM: ☐☐☐☐☐   PM: ☐☐☐☐☐
NOTES: _____
_____

LEVEL OF SLEEP AM: ☐☐☐☐☐   PM: ☐☐☐☐☐
NOTES: _____
_____

Are you noticing anything different today?
_____
_____

What is your ongoing or new goal for success in caregiving and helping your loved one to age gracefully and in a way that first their individual need and disposition?
_____
_____
_____

What were your challenges and triumphs today?
_____
_____

Do you have any questions or concerns to reach out about?
_____
_____

DATE:

TOILET / DIAPER

TIME	RESULT	
:	wet	b.m.
:	wet	b.m.
:	wet	b.m.
:	wet	b.m.
:	wet	b.m.
:	wet	b.m.
:	wet	b.m.

MEALS / FEEDINGS

TIME	AMOUNT
:	
:	
:	
:	
:	
:	
:	

PERSONAL CARE

☐ Shower ☐ Bed Bath ☐ Brush Hair ☐ Teeth

PHYSICAL THERAPY

☐ Back ☐ Neck ☐ Shoulders
☐ Arms ☐ Hands ☐ Legs ☐ Feet
☐ Speech Therapy

SPECIAL CARE

MEDICINE	DOSAGE	TIME	MEDICINE	DOSAGE	TIME
		:			:
		:			:
		:			:
		:			:
		:			:
		:			:

BLOOD PRESSURE

SYSTOLIC	DIASTOLIC	TIME
		:
		:
		:
		:
		:
		:

ACTIVITIES

ACTIVITY	LENGTH

SUPPLIES NEEDED

NOTES

LEVEL OF HAPPINESS   AM: ☐☐☐☐   PM: ☐☐☐☐
NOTES: _____
_____

LEVEL OF ENGAGEMENT   AM: ☐☐☐☐   PM: ☐☐☐☐
NOTES: _____
_____

LEVEL OF DISCOMFORT   AM: ☐☐☐☐   PM: ☐☐☐☐
NOTES: _____
_____

LEVEL OF SLEEP   AM: ☐☐☐☐   PM: ☐☐☐☐
NOTES: _____
_____

Are you noticing anything different today?
_____
_____

What is your ongoing or new goal for success in caregiving and helping your loved one to age gracefully and in a way that first their individual need and disposition?
_____
_____
_____

What were your challenges and triumphs today?
_____
_____

Do you have any questions or concerns to reach out about?
_____
_____

DATE:

TOILET / DIAPER

TIME	RESULT	
:	wet	b.m.
:	wet	b.m.
:	wet	b.m.
:	wet	b.m.
:	wet	b.m.
:	wet	b.m.
:	wet	b.m.

MEALS / FEEDINGS

TIME	AMOUNT
:	
:	
:	
:	
:	
:	
:	

PERSONAL CARE

☐ Shower ☐ Bed Bath ☐ Brush Hair ☐ Teeth

PHYSICAL THERAPY

☐ Back ☐ Neck ☐ Shoulders
☐ Arms ☐ Hands ☐ Legs ☐ Feet
☐ Speech Therapy

SPECIAL CARE

MEDICINE	DOSAGE	TIME	MEDICINE	DOSAGE	TIME
		:			:
		:			:
		:			:
		:			:
		:			:
		:			:

BLOOD PRESSURE

SYSTOLIC	DIASTOLIC	TIME
		:
		:
		:
		:
		:
		:

ACTIVITIES

ACTIVITY	LENGTH

SUPPLIES NEEDED

NOTES

LEVEL OF HAPPINESS   AM: ☐☐☐☐☐   PM: ☐☐☐☐☐

NOTES: _____

_____

LEVEL OF ENGAGEMENT   AM: ☐☐☐☐☐   PM: ☐☐☐☐☐

NOTES: _____

_____

LEVEL OF DISCOMFORT   AM: ☐☐☐☐☐   PM: ☐☐☐☐☐

NOTES: _____

_____

LEVEL OF SLEEP   AM: ☐☐☐☐☐   PM: ☐☐☐☐☐

NOTES: _____

_____

Are you noticing anything different today?

_____

_____

What is your ongoing or new goal for success in caregiving and helping your loved one to age gracefully and in a way that first their individual need and disposition?

_____

_____

_____

What were your challenges and triumphs today?

_____

_____

Do you have any questions or concerns to reach out about?

_____

_____

DATE:

TOILET / DIAPER

TIME	RESULT	
:	wet	b.m.
:	wet	b.m.
:	wet	b.m.
:	wet	b.m.
:	wet	b.m.
:	wet	b.m.
:	wet	b.m.

MEALS / FEEDINGS

TIME	AMOUNT
:	
:	
:	
:	
:	
:	
:	

PERSONAL CARE

☐ Shower ☐ Bed Bath ☐ Brush Hair ☐ Teeth

PHYSICAL THERAPY

☐ Back ☐ Neck ☐ Shoulders
☐ Arms ☐ Hands ☐ Legs ☐ Feet
☐ Speech Therapy

SPECIAL CARE

MEDICINE	DOSAGE	TIME	MEDICINE	DOSAGE	TIME
		:			:
		:			:
		:			:
		:			:
		:			:
		:			:

BLOOD PRESSURE

SYSTOLIC	DIASTOLIC	TIME
		:
		:
		:
		:
		:
		:

ACTIVITIES

ACTIVITY	LENGTH

SUPPLIES NEEDED

NOTES

LEVEL OF HAPPINESS AM: ☐☐☐☐   PM: ☐☐☐☐
NOTES: _____
_____

LEVEL OF ENGAGEMENT AM: ☐☐☐☐   PM: ☐☐☐☐
NOTES: _____
_____

LEVEL OF DISCOMFORT AM: ☐☐☐☐   PM: ☐☐☐☐
NOTES: _____
_____

LEVEL OF SLEEP AM: ☐☐☐☐   PM: ☐☐☐☐
NOTES: _____
_____

Are you noticing anything different today?
_____
_____

What is your ongoing or new goal for success in caregiving and helping your loved one to age gracefully and in a way that first their individual need and disposition?
_____
_____
_____

What were your challenges and triumphs today?
_____
_____

Do you have any questions or concerns to reach out about?
_____
_____

DATE:

TOILET / DIAPER

TIME	RESULT	
:	wet	b.m.
:	wet	b.m.
:	wet	b.m.
:	wet	b.m.
:	wet	b.m.
:	wet	b.m.
:	wet	b.m.

MEALS / FEEDINGS

TIME	AMOUNT
:	
:	
:	
:	
:	
:	
:	

PERSONAL CARE

☐ Shower ☐ Bed Bath ☐ Brush Hair ☐ Teeth

PHYSICAL THERAPY

☐ Back ☐ Neck ☐ Shoulders
☐ Arms ☐ Hands ☐ Legs ☐ Feet
☐ Speech Therapy

SPECIAL CARE

MEDICINE	DOSAGE	TIME	MEDICINE	DOSAGE	TIME
		:			:
		:			:
		:			:
		:			:
		:			:
		:			:

BLOOD PRESSURE

SYSTOLIC	DIASTOLIC	TIME
		:
		:
		:
		:
		:
		:

ACTIVITIES

ACTIVITY	LENGTH

SUPPLIES NEEDED

NOTES

LEVEL OF HAPPINESS AM: ☐☐☐☐ PM: ☐☐☐☐
NOTES: _____
_____

LEVEL OF ENGAGEMENT AM: ☐☐☐☐ PM: ☐☐☐☐
NOTES: _____
_____

LEVEL OF DISCOMFORT AM: ☐☐☐☐ PM: ☐☐☐☐
NOTES: _____
_____

LEVEL OF SLEEP AM: ☐☐☐☐ PM: ☐☐☐☐
NOTES: _____
_____

Are you noticing anything different today?
_____
_____

What is your ongoing or new goal for success in caregiving and helping your loved one to age gracefully and in a way that first their individual need and disposition?
_____
_____
_____

What were your challenges and triumphs today?
_____
_____

Do you have any questions or concerns to reach out about?
_____
_____

DATE: _____

TOILET / DIAPER

TIME	RESULT	
:	wet	b.m.
:	wet	b.m.
:	wet	b.m.
:	wet	b.m.
:	wet	b.m.
:	wet	b.m.
:	wet	b.m.

MEALS / FEEDINGS

TIME	AMOUNT
:	
:	
:	
:	
:	
:	
:	

PERSONAL CARE

☐ Shower   ☐ Bed Bath   ☐ Brush Hair   ☐ Teeth

PHYSICAL THERAPY

☐ Back   ☐ Neck   ☐ Shoulders
☐ Arms   ☐ Hands   ☐ Legs   ☐ Feet
☐ Speech Therapy

SPECIAL CARE

MEDICINE	DOSAGE	TIME	MEDICINE	DOSAGE	TIME
		:			:
		:			:
		:			:
		:			:
		:			:
		:			:

BLOOD PRESSURE

SYSTOLIC	DIASTOLIC	TIME
		:
		:
		:
		:
		:
		:

ACTIVITIES

ACTIVITY	LENGTH

SUPPLIES NEEDED

NOTES

LEVEL OF HAPPINESS AM: ☐☐☐☐☐   PM: ☐☐☐☐☐
NOTES: _____
_____

LEVEL OF ENGAGEMENT AM: ☐☐☐☐☐   PM: ☐☐☐☐☐
NOTES: _____
_____

LEVEL OF DISCOMFORT AM: ☐☐☐☐☐   PM: ☐☐☐☐☐
NOTES: _____
_____

LEVEL OF SLEEP AM: ☐☐☐☐☐   PM: ☐☐☐☐☐
NOTES: _____
_____

Are you noticing anything different today?
_____
_____

What is your ongoing or new goal for success in caregiving and helping your loved one to age gracefully and in a way that first their individual need and disposition?
_____
_____
_____

What were your challenges and triumphs today?
_____
_____

Do you have any questions or concerns to reach out about?
_____
_____

DATE:

TOILET / DIAPER

TIME	RESULT	
:	wet	b.m.
:	wet	b.m.
:	wet	b.m.
:	wet	b.m.
:	wet	b.m.
:	wet	b.m.
:	wet	b.m.

MEALS / FEEDINGS

TIME	AMOUNT
:	
:	
:	
:	
:	
:	
:	

PERSONAL CARE

☐ Shower ☐ Bed Bath ☐ Brush Hair ☐ Teeth

PHYSICAL THERAPY

☐ Back ☐ Neck ☐ Shoulders
☐ Arms ☐ Hands ☐ Legs ☐ Feet
☐ Speech Therapy

SPECIAL CARE

MEDICINE	DOSAGE	TIME	MEDICINE	DOSAGE	TIME
		:			:
		:			:
		:			:
		:			:
		:			:
		:			:

BLOOD PRESSURE

SYSTOLIC	DIASTOLIC	TIME
		:
		:
		:
		:
		:
		:

ACTIVITIES

ACTIVITY	LENGTH

SUPPLIES NEEDED

NOTES

LEVEL OF HAPPINESS   AM: ☐☐☐☐   PM: ☐☐☐☐
NOTES: _____
_____

LEVEL OF ENGAGEMENT   AM: ☐☐☐☐   PM: ☐☐☐☐
NOTES: _____
_____

LEVEL OF DISCOMFORT   AM: ☐☐☐☐   PM: ☐☐☐☐
NOTES: _____
_____

LEVEL OF SLEEP   AM: ☐☐☐☐   PM: ☐☐☐☐
NOTES: _____
_____

Are you noticing anything different today?
_____
_____

What is your ongoing or new goal for success in caregiving and helping your loved one to age gracefully and in a way that first their individual need and disposition?
_____
_____
_____

What were your challenges and triumphs today?
_____
_____

Do you have any questions or concerns to reach out about?
_____
_____

DATE:

TOILET / DIAPER

TIME	RESULT	
:	wet	b.m.
:	wet	b.m.
:	wet	b.m.
:	wet	b.m.
:	wet	b.m.
:	wet	b.m.
:	wet	b.m.

MEALS / FEEDINGS

TIME	AMOUNT
:	
:	
:	
:	
:	
:	
:	

PERSONAL CARE

☐ Shower ☐ Bed Bath ☐ Brush Hair ☐ Teeth

PHYSICAL THERAPY

☐ Back ☐ Neck ☐ Shoulders
☐ Arms ☐ Hands ☐ Legs ☐ Feet
☐ Speech Therapy

SPECIAL CARE

MEDICINE	DOSAGE	TIME	MEDICINE	DOSAGE	TIME
		:			:
		:			:
		:			:
		:			:
		:			:
		:			:

BLOOD PRESSURE

SYSTOLIC	DIASTOLIC	TIME
		:
		:
		:
		:
		:
		:

ACTIVITIES

ACTIVITY	LENGTH

SUPPLIES NEEDED

NOTES

LEVEL OF HAPPINESS AM: ☐☐☐☐ PM: ☐☐☐☐
NOTES: _____
_____

LEVEL OF ENGAGEMENT AM: ☐☐☐☐ PM: ☐☐☐☐
NOTES: _____
_____

LEVEL OF DISCOMFORT AM: ☐☐☐☐ PM: ☐☐☐☐
NOTES: _____
_____

LEVEL OF SLEEP AM: ☐☐☐☐ PM: ☐☐☐☐
NOTES: _____
_____

Are you noticing anything different today?
_____
_____

What is your ongoing or new goal for success in caregiving and helping your loved one to age gracefully and in a way that first their individual need and disposition?
_____
_____
_____

What were your challenges and triumphs today?
_____
_____

Do you have any questions or concerns to reach out about?
_____
_____

DATE: _____

TOILET / DIAPER

TIME	RESULT	
:	wet	b.m.
:	wet	b.m.
:	wet	b.m.
:	wet	b.m.
:	wet	b.m.
:	wet	b.m.
:	wet	b.m.

MEALS / FEEDINGS

TIME	AMOUNT
:	
:	
:	
:	
:	
:	
:	

PERSONAL CARE

☐ Shower ☐ Bed Bath ☐ Brush Hair ☐ Teeth

PHYSICAL THERAPY

☐ Back ☐ Neck ☐ Shoulders
☐ Arms ☐ Hands ☐ Legs ☐ Feet
☐ Speech Therapy

SPECIAL CARE

MEDICINE	DOSAGE	TIME	MEDICINE	DOSAGE	TIME
		:			:
		:			:
		:			:
		:			:
		:			:
		:			:

BLOOD PRESSURE

SYSTOLIC	DIASTOLIC	TIME
		:
		:
		:
		:
		:
		:

ACTIVITIES

ACTIVITY	LENGTH

SUPPLIES NEEDED

NOTES

LEVEL OF HAPPINESS AM: ☐☐☐☐☐ PM: ☐☐☐☐☐
NOTES: _____
_____

LEVEL OF ENGAGEMENT AM: ☐☐☐☐☐ PM: ☐☐☐☐☐
NOTES: _____
_____

LEVEL OF DISCOMFORT AM: ☐☐☐☐☐ PM: ☐☐☐☐☐
NOTES: _____
_____

LEVEL OF SLEEP AM: ☐☐☐☐☐ PM: ☐☐☐☐☐
NOTES: _____
_____

Are you noticing anything different today?
_____
_____

What is your ongoing or new goal for success in caregiving and helping your loved one to age gracefully and in a way that first their individual need and disposition?
_____
_____
_____

What were your challenges and triumphs today?
_____
_____

Do you have any questions or concerns to reach out about?
_____
_____

DATE:

TOILET / DIAPER

TIME	RESULT	
:	wet	b.m.
:	wet	b.m.
:	wet	b.m.
:	wet	b.m.
:	wet	b.m.
:	wet	b.m.
:	wet	b.m.

MEALS / FEEDINGS

TIME	AMOUNT
:	
:	
:	
:	
:	
:	
:	

PERSONAL CARE

☐ Shower ☐ Bed Bath ☐ Brush Hair ☐ Teeth

PHYSICAL THERAPY

☐ Back   ☐ Neck   ☐ Shoulders
☐ Arms   ☐ Hands   ☐ Legs   ☐ Feet
☐ Speech Therapy

SPECIAL CARE

MEDICINE	DOSAGE	TIME	MEDICINE	DOSAGE	TIME
		:			:
		:			:
		:			:
		:			:
		:			:
		:			:

BLOOD PRESSURE

SYSTOLIC	DIASTOLIC	TIME
		:
		:
		:
		:
		:
		:

ACTIVITIES

ACTIVITY	LENGTH

SUPPLIES NEEDED

NOTES

LEVEL OF HAPPINESS　　AM: ☐☐☐☐☐　　PM: ☐☐☐☐☐
NOTES: _____
_____

LEVEL OF ENGAGEMENT　AM: ☐☐☐☐☐　　PM: ☐☐☐☐☐
NOTES: _____
_____

LEVEL OF DISCOMFORT　AM: ☐☐☐☐☐　　PM: ☐☐☐☐☐
NOTES: _____
_____

LEVEL OF SLEEP　　　　AM: ☐☐☐☐☐　　PM: ☐☐☐☐☐
NOTES: _____
_____

Are you noticing anything different today?
_____
_____

What is your ongoing or new goal for success in caregiving and helping your loved one to age gracefully and in a way that first their individual need and disposition?
_____
_____
_____

What were your challenges and triumphs today?
_____
_____

Do you have any questions or concerns to reach out about?
_____
_____

DATE:

TOILET / DIAPER

TIME	RESULT	
:	wet	b.m.
:	wet	b.m.
:	wet	b.m.
:	wet	b.m.
:	wet	b.m.
:	wet	b.m.
:	wet	b.m.

MEALS / FEEDINGS

TIME	AMOUNT
:	
:	
:	
:	
:	
:	
:	

PERSONAL CARE

☐ Shower ☐ Bed Bath ☐ Brush Hair ☐ Teeth

PHYSICAL THERAPY

☐ Back ☐ Neck ☐ Shoulders
☐ Arms ☐ Hands ☐ Legs ☐ Feet
☐ Speech Therapy

SPECIAL CARE

MEDICINE	DOSAGE	TIME	MEDICINE	DOSAGE	TIME
		:			:
		:			:
		:			:
		:			:
		:			:
		:			:

BLOOD PRESSURE

SYSTOLIC	DIASTOLIC	TIME
		:
		:
		:
		:
		:
		:

ACTIVITIES

ACTIVITY	LENGTH

SUPPLIES NEEDED

NOTES

LEVEL OF HAPPINESS   AM: ☐☐☐☐   PM: ☐☐☐☐
NOTES: _____
_____

LEVEL OF ENGAGEMENT   AM: ☐☐☐☐   PM: ☐☐☐☐
NOTES: _____
_____

LEVEL OF DISCOMFORT   AM: ☐☐☐☐   PM: ☐☐☐☐
NOTES: _____
_____

LEVEL OF SLEEP   AM: ☐☐☐☐   PM: ☐☐☐☐
NOTES: _____
_____

Are you noticing anything different today?
_____
_____

What is your ongoing or new goal for success in caregiving and helping your loved one to age gracefully and in a way that first their individual need and disposition?
_____
_____
_____

What were your challenges and triumphs today?
_____
_____

Do you have any questions or concerns to reach out about?
_____
_____

DATE:

TOILET / DIAPER

TIME	RESULT	
:	wet	b.m.
:	wet	b.m.
:	wet	b.m.
:	wet	b.m.
:	wet	b.m.
:	wet	b.m.
:	wet	b.m.

MEALS / FEEDINGS

TIME	AMOUNT
:	
:	
:	
:	
:	
:	
:	

PERSONAL CARE

☐ Shower ☐ Bed Bath ☐ Brush Hair ☐ Teeth

PHYSICAL THERAPY

☐ Back   ☐ Neck   ☐ Shoulders

☐ Arms   ☐ Hands   ☐ Legs   ☐ Feet

☐ Speech Therapy

SPECIAL CARE

MEDICINE	DOSAGE	TIME	MEDICINE	DOSAGE	TIME
		:			:
		:			:
		:			:
		:			:
		:			:
		:			:

BLOOD PRESSURE

SYSTOLIC	DIASTOLIC	TIME
		:
		:
		:
		:
		:
		:

ACTIVITIES

ACTIVITY	LENGTH

SUPPLIES NEEDED

NOTES

LEVEL OF HAPPINESS   AM: ☐☐☐☐   PM: ☐☐☐☐
NOTES: _____
_____

LEVEL OF ENGAGEMENT   AM: ☐☐☐☐   PM: ☐☐☐☐
NOTES: _____
_____

LEVEL OF DISCOMFORT   AM: ☐☐☐☐   PM: ☐☐☐☐
NOTES: _____
_____

LEVEL OF SLEEP   AM: ☐☐☐☐   PM: ☐☐☐☐
NOTES: _____
_____

Are you noticing anything different today?
_____
_____

What is your ongoing or new goal for success in caregiving and helping your loved one to age gracefully and in a way that first their individual need and disposition?
_____
_____
_____

What were your challenges and triumphs today?
_____
_____

Do you have any questions or concerns to reach out about?
_____
_____

DATE:

TOILET / DIAPER

TIME	RESULT	
:	wet	b.m.
:	wet	b.m.
:	wet	b.m.
:	wet	b.m.
:	wet	b.m.
:	wet	b.m.
:	wet	b.m.

MEALS / FEEDINGS

TIME	AMOUNT
:	
:	
:	
:	
:	
:	
:	

PERSONAL CARE

☐ Shower ☐ Bed Bath ☐ Brush Hair ☐ Teeth

PHYSICAL THERAPY

☐ Back ☐ Neck ☐ Shoulders
☐ Arms ☐ Hands ☐ Legs ☐ Feet
☐ Speech Therapy

SPECIAL CARE

MEDICINE	DOSAGE	TIME	MEDICINE	DOSAGE	TIME
		:			:
		:			:
		:			:
		:			:
		:			:
		:			:

BLOOD PRESSURE

SYSTOLIC	DIASTOLIC	TIME
		:
		:
		:
		:
		:
		:

ACTIVITIES

ACTIVITY	LENGTH

SUPPLIES NEEDED

NOTES

LEVEL OF HAPPINESS   AM: ☐☐☐☐   PM: ☐☐☐☐
NOTES: _____
_____

LEVEL OF ENGAGEMENT   AM: ☐☐☐☐   PM: ☐☐☐☐
NOTES: _____
_____

LEVEL OF DISCOMFORT   AM: ☐☐☐☐   PM: ☐☐☐☐
NOTES: _____
_____

LEVEL OF SLEEP   AM: ☐☐☐☐   PM: ☐☐☐☐
NOTES: _____
_____

Are you noticing anything different today?
_____
_____

What is your ongoing or new goal for success in caregiving and helping your loved one to age gracefully and in a way that first their individual need and disposition?
_____
_____
_____

What were your challenges and triumphs today?
_____
_____

Do you have any questions or concerns to reach out about?
_____
_____

DATE:

TOILET / DIAPER

TIME	RESULT	
:	wet	b.m.
:	wet	b.m.
:	wet	b.m.
:	wet	b.m.
:	wet	b.m.
:	wet	b.m.
:	wet	b.m.

MEALS / FEEDINGS

TIME	AMOUNT
:	
:	
:	
:	
:	
:	
:	

PERSONAL CARE

☐ Shower ☐ Bed Bath ☐ Brush Hair ☐ Teeth

PHYSICAL THERAPY

☐ Back ☐ Neck ☐ Shoulders
☐ Arms ☐ Hands ☐ Legs ☐ Feet
☐ Speech Therapy

SPECIAL CARE

MEDICINE	DOSAGE	TIME	MEDICINE	DOSAGE	TIME
		:			:
		:			:
		:			:
		:			:
		:			:
		:			:

BLOOD PRESSURE

SYSTOLIC	DIASTOLIC	TIME
		:
		:
		:
		:
		:
		:

ACTIVITIES

ACTIVITY	LENGTH

SUPPLIES NEEDED

NOTES

LEVEL OF HAPPINESS   AM: ☐☐☐☐   PM: ☐☐☐☐
NOTES: _____
_____

LEVEL OF ENGAGEMENT   AM: ☐☐☐☐   PM: ☐☐☐☐
NOTES: _____
_____

LEVEL OF DISCOMFORT   AM: ☐☐☐☐   PM: ☐☐☐☐
NOTES: _____
_____

LEVEL OF SLEEP   AM: ☐☐☐☐   PM: ☐☐☐☐
NOTES: _____
_____

Are you noticing anything different today?
_____
_____

What is your ongoing or new goal for success in caregiving and helping your loved one to age gracefully and in a way that first their individual need and disposition?
_____
_____
_____

What were your challenges and triumphs today?
_____
_____

Do you have any questions or concerns to reach out about?
_____
_____

DATE:

TOILET / DIAPER

TIME	RESULT	
:	wet	b.m.
:	wet	b.m.
:	wet	b.m.
:	wet	b.m.
:	wet	b.m.
:	wet	b.m.
:	wet	b.m.

MEALS / FEEDINGS

TIME	AMOUNT
:	
:	
:	
:	
:	
:	
:	

PERSONAL CARE

☐ Shower ☐ Bed Bath ☐ Brush Hair ☐ Teeth

PHYSICAL THERAPY

☐ Back ☐ Neck ☐ Shoulders
☐ Arms ☐ Hands ☐ Legs ☐ Feet
☐ Speech Therapy

SPECIAL CARE

MEDICINE	DOSAGE	TIME	MEDICINE	DOSAGE	TIME
		:			:
		:			:
		:			:
		:			:
		:			:
		:			:

BLOOD PRESSURE

SYSTOLIC	DIASTOLIC	TIME
		:
		:
		:
		:
		:
		:

ACTIVITIES

ACTIVITY	LENGTH

SUPPLIES NEEDED

NOTES

LEVEL OF HAPPINESS   AM: ☐☐☐☐☐   PM: ☐☐☐☐☐
NOTES: _____
_____

LEVEL OF ENGAGEMENT   AM: ☐☐☐☐☐   PM: ☐☐☐☐☐
NOTES: _____
_____

LEVEL OF DISCOMFORT   AM: ☐☐☐☐☐   PM: ☐☐☐☐☐
NOTES: _____
_____

LEVEL OF SLEEP   AM: ☐☐☐☐☐   PM: ☐☐☐☐☐
NOTES: _____
_____

Are you noticing anything different today?
_____
_____

What is your ongoing or new goal for success in caregiving and helping your loved one to age gracefully and in a way that first their individual need and disposition?
_____
_____
_____

What were your challenges and triumphs today?
_____
_____

Do you have any questions or concerns to reach out about?
_____
_____

DATE:

TOILET / DIAPER

TIME	RESULT	
:	wet	b.m.
:	wet	b.m.
:	wet	b.m.
:	wet	b.m.
:	wet	b.m.
:	wet	b.m.
:	wet	b.m.

MEALS / FEEDINGS

TIME	AMOUNT
:	
:	
:	
:	
:	
:	
:	

PERSONAL CARE

☐ Shower ☐ Bed Bath ☐ Brush Hair ☐ Teeth

PHYSICAL THERAPY

☐ Back ☐ Neck ☐ Shoulders
☐ Arms ☐ Hands ☐ Legs ☐ Feet
☐ Speech Therapy

SPECIAL CARE

MEDICINE	DOSAGE	TIME	MEDICINE	DOSAGE	TIME
		:			:
		:			:
		:			:
		:			:
		:			:
		:			:

BLOOD PRESSURE

SYSTOLIC	DIASTOLIC	TIME
		:
		:
		:
		:
		:
		:

ACTIVITIES

ACTIVITY	LENGTH

SUPPLIES NEEDED

NOTES

LEVEL OF HAPPINESS AM: ☐☐☐☐☐   PM: ☐☐☐☐☐
NOTES: _____
_____

LEVEL OF ENGAGEMENT AM: ☐☐☐☐☐   PM: ☐☐☐☐☐
NOTES: _____
_____

LEVEL OF DISCOMFORT AM: ☐☐☐☐☐   PM: ☐☐☐☐☐
NOTES: _____
_____

LEVEL OF SLEEP AM: ☐☐☐☐☐   PM: ☐☐☐☐☐
NOTES: _____
_____

Are you noticing anything different today?
_____
_____

What is your ongoing or new goal for success in caregiving and helping your loved one to age gracefully and in a way that first their individual need and disposition?
_____
_____
_____

What were your challenges and triumphs today?
_____
_____

Do you have any questions or concerns to reach out about?
_____
_____

DATE:

TOILET / DIAPER

TIME	RESULT	
:	wet	b.m.
:	wet	b.m.
:	wet	b.m.
:	wet	b.m.
:	wet	b.m.
:	wet	b.m.
:	wet	b.m.

MEALS / FEEDINGS

TIME	AMOUNT
:	
:	
:	
:	
:	
:	
:	

PERSONAL CARE

☐ Shower ☐ Bed Bath ☐ Brush Hair ☐ Teeth

PHYSICAL THERAPY

☐ Back ☐ Neck ☐ Shoulders
☐ Arms ☐ Hands ☐ Legs ☐ Feet
☐ Speech Therapy

SPECIAL CARE

MEDICINE	DOSAGE	TIME	MEDICINE	DOSAGE	TIME
		:			:
		:			:
		:			:
		:			:
		:			:
		:			:

BLOOD PRESSURE

SYSTOLIC	DIASTOLIC	TIME
		:
		:
		:
		:
		:
		:

ACTIVITIES

ACTIVITY	LENGTH

SUPPLIES NEEDED

NOTES

LEVEL OF HAPPINESS   AM: ☐☐☐☐☐   PM: ☐☐☐☐☐
NOTES: _____
_____

LEVEL OF ENGAGEMENT   AM: ☐☐☐☐☐   PM: ☐☐☐☐☐
NOTES: _____
_____

LEVEL OF DISCOMFORT   AM: ☐☐☐☐☐   PM: ☐☐☐☐☐
NOTES: _____
_____

LEVEL OF SLEEP   AM: ☐☐☐☐☐   PM: ☐☐☐☐☐
NOTES: _____
_____

Are you noticing anything different today?
_____
_____

What is your ongoing or new goal for success in caregiving and helping your loved one to age gracefully and in a way that first their individual need and disposition?
_____
_____
_____

What were your challenges and triumphs today?
_____
_____

Do you have any questions or concerns to reach out about?
_____
_____

DATE:

TOILET / DIAPER

TIME	RESULT	
:	wet	b.m.
:	wet	b.m.
:	wet	b.m.
:	wet	b.m.
:	wet	b.m.
:	wet	b.m.
:	wet	b.m.

MEALS / FEEDINGS

TIME	AMOUNT
:	
:	
:	
:	
:	
:	
:	

PERSONAL CARE

☐ Shower ☐ Bed Bath ☐ Brush Hair ☐ Teeth

PHYSICAL THERAPY

☐ Back ☐ Neck ☐ Shoulders
☐ Arms ☐ Hands ☐ Legs ☐ Feet
☐ Speech Therapy

SPECIAL CARE

MEDICINE	DOSAGE	TIME	MEDICINE	DOSAGE	TIME
		:			:
		:			:
		:			:
		:			:
		:			:
		:			:

BLOOD PRESSURE

SYSTOLIC	DIASTOLIC	TIME
		:
		:
		:
		:
		:
		:

ACTIVITIES

ACTIVITY	LENGTH

SUPPLIES NEEDED

NOTES

LEVEL OF HAPPINESS   AM: ☐☐☐☐☐   PM: ☐☐☐☐☐
NOTES: _____
_____

LEVEL OF ENGAGEMENT   AM: ☐☐☐☐☐   PM: ☐☐☐☐☐
NOTES: _____
_____

LEVEL OF DISCOMFORT   AM: ☐☐☐☐☐   PM: ☐☐☐☐☐
NOTES: _____
_____

LEVEL OF SLEEP   AM: ☐☐☐☐☐   PM: ☐☐☐☐☐
NOTES: _____
_____

Are you noticing anything different today?
_____
_____

What is your ongoing or new goal for success in caregiving and helping your loved one to age gracefully and in a way that first their individual need and disposition?
_____
_____
_____

What were your challenges and triumphs today?
_____
_____

Do you have any questions or concerns to reach out about?
_____
_____

DATE: _____

TOILET / DIAPER

TIME	RESULT	
:	wet	b.m.
:	wet	b.m.
:	wet	b.m.
:	wet	b.m.
:	wet	b.m.
:	wet	b.m.
:	wet	b.m.

MEALS / FEEDINGS

TIME	AMOUNT
:	
:	
:	
:	
:	
:	
:	

PERSONAL CARE

☐ Shower ☐ Bed Bath ☐ Brush Hair ☐ Teeth

PHYSICAL THERAPY

☐ Back ☐ Neck ☐ Shoulders
☐ Arms ☐ Hands ☐ Legs ☐ Feet
☐ Speech Therapy

SPECIAL CARE

MEDICINE	DOSAGE	TIME	MEDICINE	DOSAGE	TIME
		:			:
		:			:
		:			:
		:			:
		:			:
		:			:

BLOOD PRESSURE

SYSTOLIC	DIASTOLIC	TIME
		:
		:
		:
		:
		:
		:

ACTIVITIES

ACTIVITY	LENGTH

SUPPLIES NEEDED

NOTES

LEVEL OF HAPPINESS AM: [   ][   ][   ][   ] PM: [   ][   ][   ][   ]
NOTES: _____
_____

LEVEL OF ENGAGEMENT AM: [   ][   ][   ][   ] PM: [   ][   ][   ][   ]
NOTES: _____
_____

LEVEL OF DISCOMFORT AM: [   ][   ][   ][   ] PM: [   ][   ][   ][   ]
NOTES: _____
_____

LEVEL OF SLEEP AM: [   ][   ][   ][   ] PM: [   ][   ][   ][   ]
NOTES: _____
_____

Are you noticing anything different today?
_____
_____

What is your ongoing or new goal for success in caregiving and helping your loved one to age gracefully and in a way that first their individual need and disposition?
_____
_____
_____

What were your challenges and triumphs today?
_____
_____

Do you have any questions or concerns to reach out about?
_____
_____

DATE:

TOILET / DIAPER

TIME	RESULT	
:	wet	b.m.
:	wet	b.m.
:	wet	b.m.
:	wet	b.m.
:	wet	b.m.
:	wet	b.m.
:	wet	b.m.

MEALS / FEEDINGS

TIME	AMOUNT
:	
:	
:	
:	
:	
:	
:	

PERSONAL CARE

☐ Shower ☐ Bed Bath ☐ Brush Hair ☐ Teeth

PHYSICAL THERAPY

☐ Back ☐ Neck ☐ Shoulders
☐ Arms ☐ Hands ☐ Legs ☐ Feet
☐ Speech Therapy

SPECIAL CARE

MEDICINE	DOSAGE	TIME	MEDICINE	DOSAGE	TIME
		:			:
		:			:
		:			:
		:			:
		:			:
		:			:

BLOOD PRESSURE

SYSTOLIC	DIASTOLIC	TIME
		:
		:
		:
		:
		:
		:

ACTIVITIES

ACTIVITY	LENGTH

SUPPLIES NEEDED

NOTES

LEVEL OF HAPPINESS   AM: ☐☐☐☐☐   PM: ☐☐☐☐☐
NOTES: _____
_____

LEVEL OF ENGAGEMENT   AM: ☐☐☐☐☐   PM: ☐☐☐☐☐
NOTES: _____
_____

LEVEL OF DISCOMFORT   AM: ☐☐☐☐☐   PM: ☐☐☐☐☐
NOTES: _____
_____

LEVEL OF SLEEP   AM: ☐☐☐☐☐   PM: ☐☐☐☐☐
NOTES: _____
_____

Are you noticing anything different today?
_____
_____

What is your ongoing or new goal for success in caregiving and helping your loved one to age gracefully and in a way that first their individual need and disposition?
_____
_____
_____

What were your challenges and triumphs today?
_____
_____

Do you have any questions or concerns to reach out about?
_____
_____

DATE:

TOILET / DIAPER

TIME	RESULT	
:	wet	b.m.
:	wet	b.m.
:	wet	b.m.
:	wet	b.m.
:	wet	b.m.
:	wet	b.m.
:	wet	b.m.

MEALS / FEEDINGS

TIME	AMOUNT
:	
:	
:	
:	
:	
:	
:	

PERSONAL CARE

☐ Shower ☐ Bed Bath ☐ Brush Hair ☐ Teeth

PHYSICAL THERAPY

☐ Back   ☐ Neck   ☐ Shoulders
☐ Arms   ☐ Hands   ☐ Legs   ☐ Feet
☐ Speech Therapy

SPECIAL CARE

MEDICINE	DOSAGE	TIME	MEDICINE	DOSAGE	TIME
		:			:
		:			:
		:			:
		:			:
		:			:
		:			:

BLOOD PRESSURE

SYSTOLIC	DIASTOLIC	TIME
		:
		:
		:
		:
		:
		:

ACTIVITIES

ACTIVITY	LENGTH

SUPPLIES NEEDED

NOTES

LEVEL OF HAPPINESS   AM: ▢▢▢▢▢   PM: ▢▢▢▢▢

NOTES: _____

_____

LEVEL OF ENGAGEMENT   AM: ▢▢▢▢▢   PM: ▢▢▢▢▢

NOTES: _____

_____

LEVEL OF DISCOMFORT   AM: ▢▢▢▢▢   PM: ▢▢▢▢▢

NOTES: _____

_____

LEVEL OF SLEEP   AM: ▢▢▢▢▢   PM: ▢▢▢▢▢

NOTES: _____

_____

Are you noticing anything different today?

_____

_____

What is your ongoing or new goal for success in caregiving and helping your loved one to age gracefully and in a way that first their individual need and disposition?

_____

_____

_____

What were your challenges and triumphs today?

_____

_____

Do you have any questions or concerns to reach out about?

_____

_____

DATE:

TOILET / DIAPER

TIME	RESULT	
:	wet	b.m.
:	wet	b.m.
:	wet	b.m.
:	wet	b.m.
:	wet	b.m.
:	wet	b.m.
:	wet	b.m.

MEALS / FEEDINGS

TIME	AMOUNT
:	
:	
:	
:	
:	
:	
:	

PERSONAL CARE

☐ Shower ☐ Bed Bath ☐ Brush Hair ☐ Teeth

PHYSICAL THERAPY

☐ Back ☐ Neck ☐ Shoulders
☐ Arms ☐ Hands ☐ Legs ☐ Feet
☐ Speech Therapy

SPECIAL CARE

MEDICINE	DOSAGE	TIME	MEDICINE	DOSAGE	TIME
		:			:
		:			:
		:			:
		:			:
		:			:
		:			:

BLOOD PRESSURE

SYSTOLIC	DIASTOLIC	TIME
		:
		:
		:
		:
		:
		:

ACTIVITIES

ACTIVITY	LENGTH

SUPPLIES NEEDED

NOTES

LEVEL OF HAPPINESS AM: ☐☐☐☐☐   PM: ☐☐☐☐☐
NOTES: _____
_____

LEVEL OF ENGAGEMENT AM: ☐☐☐☐☐   PM: ☐☐☐☐☐
NOTES: _____
_____

LEVEL OF DISCOMFORT AM: ☐☐☐☐☐   PM: ☐☐☐☐☐
NOTES: _____
_____

LEVEL OF SLEEP AM: ☐☐☐☐☐   PM: ☐☐☐☐☐
NOTES: _____
_____

Are you noticing anything different today?
_____
_____

What is your ongoing or new goal for success in caregiving and helping your loved one to age gracefully and in a way that first their individual need and disposition?
_____
_____
_____

What were your challenges and triumphs today?
_____
_____

Do you have any questions or concerns to reach out about?
_____
_____

DATE: _____

TOILET / DIAPER

TIME	RESULT	
:	wet	b.m.
:	wet	b.m.
:	wet	b.m.
:	wet	b.m.
:	wet	b.m.
:	wet	b.m.
:	wet	b.m.

MEALS / FEEDINGS

TIME	AMOUNT
:	
:	
:	
:	
:	
:	
:	

PERSONAL CARE

☐ Shower ☐ Bed Bath ☐ Brush Hair ☐ Teeth

PHYSICAL THERAPY

☐ Back   ☐ Neck   ☐ Shoulders
☐ Arms   ☐ Hands   ☐ Legs   ☐ Feet
☐ Speech Therapy

SPECIAL CARE

MEDICINE	DOSAGE	TIME	MEDICINE	DOSAGE	TIME
		:			:
		:			:
		:			:
		:			:
		:			:
		:			:

BLOOD PRESSURE

SYSTOLIC	DIASTOLIC	TIME
		:
		:
		:
		:
		:
		:

ACTIVITIES

ACTIVITY	LENGTH

SUPPLIES NEEDED

NOTES

LEVEL OF HAPPINESS   AM: ▭▭▭▭▭   PM: ▭▭▭▭▭
NOTES: _____
_____

LEVEL OF ENGAGEMENT   AM: ▭▭▭▭▭   PM: ▭▭▭▭▭
NOTES: _____
_____

LEVEL OF DISCOMFORT   AM: ▭▭▭▭▭   PM: ▭▭▭▭▭
NOTES: _____
_____

LEVEL OF SLEEP   AM: ▭▭▭▭▭   PM: ▭▭▭▭▭
NOTES: _____
_____

Are you noticing anything different today?
_____
_____

What is your ongoing or new goal for success in caregiving and helping your loved one to age gracefully and in a way that first their individual need and disposition?
_____
_____
_____

What were your challenges and triumphs today?
_____
_____

Do you have any questions or concerns to reach out about?
_____
_____

DATE:

TOILET / DIAPER

TIME	RESULT	
:	wet	b.m.
:	wet	b.m.
:	wet	b.m.
:	wet	b.m.
:	wet	b.m.
:	wet	b.m.
:	wet	b.m.

MEALS / FEEDINGS

TIME	AMOUNT
:	
:	
:	
:	
:	
:	
:	

PERSONAL CARE

☐ Shower ☐ Bed Bath ☐ Brush Hair ☐ Teeth

PHYSICAL THERAPY

☐ Back ☐ Neck ☐ Shoulders
☐ Arms ☐ Hands ☐ Legs ☐ Feet
☐ Speech Therapy

SPECIAL CARE

MEDICINE	DOSAGE	TIME	MEDICINE	DOSAGE	TIME
		:			:
		:			:
		:			:
		:			:
		:			:
		:			:

BLOOD PRESSURE

SYSTOLIC	DIASTOLIC	TIME
		:
		:
		:
		:
		:
		:

ACTIVITIES

ACTIVITY	LENGTH

SUPPLIES NEEDED

NOTES

LEVEL OF HAPPINESS   AM: ☐☐☐☐☐   PM: ☐☐☐☐☐

NOTES: _____

_____

LEVEL OF ENGAGEMENT   AM: ☐☐☐☐☐   PM: ☐☐☐☐☐

NOTES: _____

_____

LEVEL OF DISCOMFORT   AM: ☐☐☐☐☐   PM: ☐☐☐☐☐

NOTES: _____

_____

LEVEL OF SLEEP   AM: ☐☐☐☐☐   PM: ☐☐☐☐☐

NOTES: _____

_____

Are you noticing anything different today?

_____

_____

What is your ongoing or new goal for success in caregiving and helping your loved one to age gracefully and in a way that first their individual need and disposition?

_____

_____

_____

What were your challenges and triumphs today?

_____

_____

Do you have any questions or concerns to reach out about?

_____

_____

DATE:

TOILET / DIAPER

TIME	RESULT	
:	wet	b.m.
:	wet	b.m.
:	wet	b.m.
:	wet	b.m.
:	wet	b.m.
:	wet	b.m.
:	wet	b.m.

MEALS / FEEDINGS

TIME	AMOUNT
:	
:	
:	
:	
:	
:	
:	

PERSONAL CARE

☐ Shower ☐ Bed Bath ☐ Brush Hair ☐ Teeth

PHYSICAL THERAPY

☐ Back ☐ Neck ☐ Shoulders
☐ Arms ☐ Hands ☐ Legs ☐ Feet
☐ Speech Therapy

SPECIAL CARE

MEDICINE	DOSAGE	TIME	MEDICINE	DOSAGE	TIME
		:			:
		:			:
		:			:
		:			:
		:			:
		:			:

BLOOD PRESSURE

SYSTOLIC	DIASTOLIC	TIME
		:
		:
		:
		:
		:
		:

ACTIVITIES

ACTIVITY	LENGTH

SUPPLIES NEEDED

NOTES

LEVEL OF HAPPINESS   AM: ☐☐☐☐☐   PM: ☐☐☐☐☐
NOTES: _____
_____

LEVEL OF ENGAGEMENT   AM: ☐☐☐☐☐   PM: ☐☐☐☐☐
NOTES: _____
_____

LEVEL OF DISCOMFORT   AM: ☐☐☐☐☐   PM: ☐☐☐☐☐
NOTES: _____
_____

LEVEL OF SLEEP   AM: ☐☐☐☐☐   PM: ☐☐☐☐☐
NOTES: _____
_____

Are you noticing anything different today?
_____
_____

What is your ongoing or new goal for success in caregiving and helping your loved one to age gracefully and in a way that first their individual need and disposition?
_____
_____
_____

What were your challenges and triumphs today?
_____
_____

Do you have any questions or concerns to reach out about?
_____
_____

DATE:

TOILET / DIAPER

TIME	RESULT	
:	wet	b.m.
:	wet	b.m.
:	wet	b.m.
:	wet	b.m.
:	wet	b.m.
:	wet	b.m.
:	wet	b.m.

MEALS / FEEDINGS

TIME	AMOUNT
:	
:	
:	
:	
:	
:	
:	

PERSONAL CARE

☐ Shower ☐ Bed Bath ☐ Brush Hair ☐ Teeth

PHYSICAL THERAPY

☐ Back ☐ Neck ☐ Shoulders

☐ Arms ☐ Hands ☐ Legs ☐ Feet

☐ Speech Therapy

SPECIAL CARE

MEDICINE	DOSAGE	TIME	MEDICINE	DOSAGE	TIME
		:			:
		:			:
		:			:
		:			:
		:			:
		:			:

BLOOD PRESSURE

SYSTOLIC	DIASTOLIC	TIME
		:
		:
		:
		:
		:
		:

ACTIVITIES

ACTIVITY	LENGTH

SUPPLIES NEEDED

NOTES

LEVEL OF HAPPINESS   AM: ☐   PM: ☐
NOTES: _____
_____

LEVEL OF ENGAGEMENT   AM: ☐   PM: ☐
NOTES: _____
_____

LEVEL OF DISCOMFORT   AM: ☐   PM: ☐
NOTES: _____
_____

LEVEL OF SLEEP   AM: ☐   PM: ☐
NOTES: _____
_____

Are you noticing anything different today?
_____
_____

What is your ongoing or new goal for success in caregiving and helping your loved one to age gracefully and in a way that first their individual need and disposition?
_____
_____

What were your challenges and triumphs today?
_____
_____

Do you have any questions or concerns to reach out about?
_____
_____

DATE:

TOILET / DIAPER

TIME	RESULT	
:	wet	b.m.
:	wet	b.m.
:	wet	b.m.
:	wet	b.m.
:	wet	b.m.
:	wet	b.m.
:	wet	b.m.

MEALS / FEEDINGS

TIME	AMOUNT
:	
:	
:	
:	
:	
:	
:	

PERSONAL CARE

☐ Shower ☐ Bed Bath ☐ Brush Hair ☐ Teeth

PHYSICAL THERAPY

☐ Back ☐ Neck ☐ Shoulders
☐ Arms ☐ Hands ☐ Legs ☐ Feet
☐ Speech Therapy

SPECIAL CARE

MEDICINE	DOSAGE	TIME	MEDICINE	DOSAGE	TIME
		:			:
		:			:
		:			:
		:			:
		:			:
		:			:

BLOOD PRESSURE

SYSTOLIC	DIASTOLIC	TIME
		:
		:
		:
		:
		:
		:

ACTIVITIES

ACTIVITY	LENGTH

SUPPLIES NEEDED

NOTES

LEVEL OF HAPPINESS AM: ☐☐☐☐☐ PM: ☐☐☐☐☐
NOTES: _____
_____

LEVEL OF ENGAGEMENT AM: ☐☐☐☐☐ PM: ☐☐☐☐☐
NOTES: _____
_____

LEVEL OF DISCOMFORT AM: ☐☐☐☐☐ PM: ☐☐☐☐☐
NOTES: _____
_____

LEVEL OF SLEEP AM: ☐☐☐☐☐ PM: ☐☐☐☐☐
NOTES: _____
_____

Are you noticing anything different today?
_____
_____

What is your ongoing or new goal for success in caregiving and helping your loved one to age gracefully and in a way that first their individual need and disposition?
_____
_____
_____

What were your challenges and triumphs today?
_____
_____

Do you have any questions or concerns to reach out about?
_____
_____

DATE:

TOILET / DIAPER

TIME	RESULT	
:	wet	b.m.
:	wet	b.m.
:	wet	b.m.
:	wet	b.m.
:	wet	b.m.
:	wet	b.m.
:	wet	b.m.

MEALS / FEEDINGS

TIME	AMOUNT
:	
:	
:	
:	
:	
:	
:	

PERSONAL CARE

☐ Shower ☐ Bed Bath ☐ Brush Hair ☐ Teeth

PHYSICAL THERAPY

☐ Back ☐ Neck ☐ Shoulders
☐ Arms ☐ Hands ☐ Legs ☐ Feet
☐ Speech Therapy

SPECIAL CARE

MEDICINE	DOSAGE	TIME	MEDICINE	DOSAGE	TIME
		:			:
		:			:
		:			:
		:			:
		:			:
		:			:

BLOOD PRESSURE

SYSTOLIC	DIASTOLIC	TIME
		:
		:
		:
		:
		:
		:

ACTIVITIES

ACTIVITY	LENGTH

SUPPLIES NEEDED

NOTES

LEVEL OF HAPPINESS AM: ☐☐☐☐☐   PM: ☐☐☐☐☐
NOTES: _____
_____

LEVEL OF ENGAGEMENT AM: ☐☐☐☐☐   PM: ☐☐☐☐☐
NOTES: _____
_____

LEVEL OF DISCOMFORT AM: ☐☐☐☐☐   PM: ☐☐☐☐☐
NOTES: _____
_____

LEVEL OF SLEEP AM: ☐☐☐☐☐   PM: ☐☐☐☐☐
NOTES: _____
_____

Are you noticing anything different today?
_____
_____

What is your ongoing or new goal for success in caregiving and helping your loved one to age gracefully and in a way that first their individual need and disposition?
_____
_____
_____

What were your challenges and triumphs today?
_____
_____

Do you have any questions or concerns to reach out about?
_____
_____

DATE:

TOILET / DIAPER

TIME	RESULT	
:	wet	b.m.
:	wet	b.m.
:	wet	b.m.
:	wet	b.m.
:	wet	b.m.
:	wet	b.m.
:	wet	b.m.

MEALS / FEEDINGS

TIME	AMOUNT
:	
:	
:	
:	
:	
:	
:	

PERSONAL CARE

☐ Shower ☐ Bed Bath ☐ Brush Hair ☐ Teeth

PHYSICAL THERAPY

☐ Back ☐ Neck ☐ Shoulders
☐ Arms ☐ Hands ☐ Legs ☐ Feet
☐ Speech Therapy

SPECIAL CARE

MEDICINE	DOSAGE	TIME	MEDICINE	DOSAGE	TIME
		:			:
		:			:
		:			:
		:			:
		:			:
		:			:

BLOOD PRESSURE

SYSTOLIC	DIASTOLIC	TIME
		:
		:
		:
		:
		:
		:

ACTIVITIES

ACTIVITY	LENGTH

SUPPLIES NEEDED

NOTES

LEVEL OF HAPPINESS AM: ☐☐☐☐ PM: ☐☐☐☐
NOTES: _____
_____

LEVEL OF ENGAGEMENT AM: ☐☐☐☐ PM: ☐☐☐☐
NOTES: _____
_____

LEVEL OF DISCOMFORT AM: ☐☐☐☐ PM: ☐☐☐☐
NOTES: _____
_____

LEVEL OF SLEEP AM: ☐☐☐☐ PM: ☐☐☐☐
NOTES: _____
_____

Are you noticing anything different today?
_____
_____

What is your ongoing or new goal for success in caregiving and helping your loved one to age gracefully and in a way that first their individual need and disposition?
_____
_____
_____

What were your challenges and triumphs today?
_____
_____

Do you have any questions or concerns to reach out about?
_____
_____

DATE:

TOILET / DIAPER

TIME	RESULT	
:	wet	b.m.
:	wet	b.m.
:	wet	b.m.
:	wet	b.m.
:	wet	b.m.
:	wet	b.m.
:	wet	b.m.

MEALS / FEEDINGS

TIME	AMOUNT
:	
:	
:	
:	
:	
:	
:	

PERSONAL CARE

☐ Shower ☐ Bed Bath ☐ Brush Hair ☐ Teeth

PHYSICAL THERAPY

☐ Back ☐ Neck ☐ Shoulders

☐ Arms ☐ Hands ☐ Legs ☐ Feet

☐ Speech Therapy

SPECIAL CARE

MEDICINE	DOSAGE	TIME	MEDICINE	DOSAGE	TIME
		:			:
		:			:
		:			:
		:			:
		:			:
		:			:

BLOOD PRESSURE

SYSTOLIC	DIASTOLIC	TIME
		:
		:
		:
		:
		:
		:

ACTIVITIES

ACTIVITY	LENGTH

SUPPLIES NEEDED

NOTES

LEVEL OF HAPPINESS AM: ☐☐☐☐☐ PM: ☐☐☐☐☐
NOTES: _____
_____

LEVEL OF ENGAGEMENT AM: ☐☐☐☐☐ PM: ☐☐☐☐☐
NOTES: _____
_____

LEVEL OF DISCOMFORT AM: ☐☐☐☐☐ PM: ☐☐☐☐☐
NOTES: _____
_____

LEVEL OF SLEEP AM: ☐☐☐☐☐ PM: ☐☐☐☐☐
NOTES: _____
_____

Are you noticing anything different today?
_____
_____

What is your ongoing or new goal for success in caregiving and helping your loved one to age gracefully and in a way that first their individual need and disposition?
_____
_____
_____

What were your challenges and triumphs today?
_____
_____

Do you have any questions or concerns to reach out about?
_____
_____

DATE:

TOILET / DIAPER

TIME	RESULT	
:	wet	b.m.
:	wet	b.m.
:	wet	b.m.
:	wet	b.m.
:	wet	b.m.
:	wet	b.m.
:	wet	b.m.

MEALS / FEEDINGS

TIME	AMOUNT
:	
:	
:	
:	
:	
:	
:	

PERSONAL CARE

☐ Shower ☐ Bed Bath ☐ Brush Hair ☐ Teeth

PHYSICAL THERAPY

☐ Back ☐ Neck ☐ Shoulders
☐ Arms ☐ Hands ☐ Legs ☐ Feet
☐ Speech Therapy

SPECIAL CARE

MEDICINE	DOSAGE	TIME	MEDICINE	DOSAGE	TIME
		:			:
		:			:
		:			:
		:			:
		:			:
		:			:

BLOOD PRESSURE

SYSTOLIC	DIASTOLIC	TIME
		:
		:
		:
		:
		:
		:

ACTIVITIES

ACTIVITY	LENGTH

SUPPLIES NEEDED

NOTES

LEVEL OF HAPPINESS AM: [ ][ ][ ][ ][ ]   PM: [ ][ ][ ][ ][ ]
NOTES: _____
_____

LEVEL OF ENGAGEMENT AM: [ ][ ][ ][ ][ ]   PM: [ ][ ][ ][ ][ ]
NOTES: _____
_____

LEVEL OF DISCOMFORT AM: [ ][ ][ ][ ][ ]   PM: [ ][ ][ ][ ][ ]
NOTES: _____
_____

LEVEL OF SLEEP AM: [ ][ ][ ][ ][ ]   PM: [ ][ ][ ][ ][ ]
NOTES: _____
_____

Are you noticing anything different today?
_____
_____

What is your ongoing or new goal for success in caregiving and helping your loved one to age gracefully and in a way that first their individual need and disposition?
_____
_____
_____

What were your challenges and triumphs today?
_____
_____

Do you have any questions or concerns to reach out about?
_____
_____

DATE:

TOILET / DIAPER

TIME	RESULT	
:	wet	b.m.
:	wet	b.m.
:	wet	b.m.
:	wet	b.m.
:	wet	b.m.
:	wet	b.m.
:	wet	b.m.

MEALS / FEEDINGS

TIME	AMOUNT
:	
:	
:	
:	
:	
:	
:	

PERSONAL CARE

☐ Shower ☐ Bed Bath ☐ Brush Hair ☐ Teeth

PHYSICAL THERAPY

☐ Back ☐ Neck ☐ Shoulders
☐ Arms ☐ Hands ☐ Legs ☐ Feet
☐ Speech Therapy

SPECIAL CARE

MEDICINE	DOSAGE	TIME	MEDICINE	DOSAGE	TIME
		:			:
		:			:
		:			:
		:			:
		:			:
		:			:

BLOOD PRESSURE

SYSTOLIC	DIASTOLIC	TIME
		:
		:
		:
		:
		:
		:

ACTIVITIES

ACTIVITY	LENGTH

SUPPLIES NEEDED

NOTES

LEVEL OF HAPPINESS   AM: ☐☐☐☐   PM: ☐☐☐☐
NOTES: _____
_____

LEVEL OF ENGAGEMENT   AM: ☐☐☐☐   PM: ☐☐☐☐
NOTES: _____
_____

LEVEL OF DISCOMFORT   AM: ☐☐☐☐   PM: ☐☐☐☐
NOTES: _____
_____

LEVEL OF SLEEP   AM: ☐☐☐☐   PM: ☐☐☐☐
NOTES: _____
_____

Are you noticing anything different today?
_____
_____

What is your ongoing or new goal for success in caregiving and helping your loved one to age gracefully and in a way that first their individual need and disposition?
_____
_____
_____

What were your challenges and triumphs today?
_____
_____

Do you have any questions or concerns to reach out about?
_____
_____

DATE:

TOILET / DIAPER

TIME	RESULT	
:	wet	b.m.
:	wet	b.m.
:	wet	b.m.
:	wet	b.m.
:	wet	b.m.
:	wet	b.m.
:	wet	b.m.

MEALS / FEEDINGS

TIME	AMOUNT
:	
:	
:	
:	
:	
:	
:	

PERSONAL CARE

☐ Shower ☐ Bed Bath ☐ Brush Hair ☐ Teeth

PHYSICAL THERAPY

☐ Back ☐ Neck ☐ Shoulders
☐ Arms ☐ Hands ☐ Legs ☐ Feet
☐ Speech Therapy

SPECIAL CARE

MEDICINE	DOSAGE	TIME	MEDICINE	DOSAGE	TIME
		:			:
		:			:
		:			:
		:			:
		:			:
		:			:

BLOOD PRESSURE

SYSTOLIC	DIASTOLIC	TIME
		:
		:
		:
		:
		:
		:

ACTIVITIES

ACTIVITY	LENGTH

SUPPLIES NEEDED

NOTES

LEVEL OF HAPPINESS   AM: ☐☐☐☐   PM: ☐☐☐☐
NOTES: _____
_____

LEVEL OF ENGAGEMENT   AM: ☐☐☐☐   PM: ☐☐☐☐
NOTES: _____
_____

LEVEL OF DISCOMFORT   AM: ☐☐☐☐   PM: ☐☐☐☐
NOTES: _____
_____

LEVEL OF SLEEP   AM: ☐☐☐☐   PM: ☐☐☐☐
NOTES: _____
_____

Are you noticing anything different today?
_____
_____

What is your ongoing or new goal for success in caregiving and helping your loved one to age gracefully and in a way that first their individual need and disposition?
_____
_____
_____

What were your challenges and triumphs today?
_____
_____

Do you have any questions or concerns to reach out about?
_____
_____

DATE:

TOILET / DIAPER

TIME	RESULT	
:	wet	b.m.
:	wet	b.m.
:	wet	b.m.
:	wet	b.m.
:	wet	b.m.
:	wet	b.m.
:	wet	b.m.

MEALS / FEEDINGS

TIME	AMOUNT
:	
:	
:	
:	
:	
:	
:	

PERSONAL CARE

☐ Shower ☐ Bed Bath ☐ Brush Hair ☐ Teeth

PHYSICAL THERAPY

☐ Back ☐ Neck ☐ Shoulders
☐ Arms ☐ Hands ☐ Legs ☐ Feet
☐ Speech Therapy

SPECIAL CARE

MEDICINE	DOSAGE	TIME	MEDICINE	DOSAGE	TIME
		:			:
		:			:
		:			:
		:			:
		:			:
		:			:

BLOOD PRESSURE

SYSTOLIC	DIASTOLIC	TIME
		:
		:
		:
		:
		:
		:

ACTIVITIES

ACTIVITY	LENGTH

SUPPLIES NEEDED

NOTES

LEVEL OF HAPPINESS AM: ☐☐☐☐ PM: ☐☐☐☐
NOTES: _____
_____

LEVEL OF ENGAGEMENT AM: ☐☐☐☐ PM: ☐☐☐☐
NOTES: _____
_____

LEVEL OF DISCOMFORT AM: ☐☐☐☐ PM: ☐☐☐☐
NOTES: _____
_____

LEVEL OF SLEEP AM: ☐☐☐☐ PM: ☐☐☐☐
NOTES: _____
_____

Are you noticing anything different today?
_____
_____

What is your ongoing or new goal for success in caregiving and helping your loved one to age gracefully and in a way that first their individual need and disposition?
_____
_____
_____

What were your challenges and triumphs today?
_____
_____

Do you have any questions or concerns to reach out about?
_____
_____

DATE: _____

TOILET / DIAPER

TIME	RESULT	
:	wet	b.m.
:	wet	b.m.
:	wet	b.m.
:	wet	b.m.
:	wet	b.m.
:	wet	b.m.
:	wet	b.m.

MEALS / FEEDINGS

TIME	AMOUNT
:	
:	
:	
:	
:	
:	
:	

PERSONAL CARE

☐ Shower ☐ Bed Bath ☐ Brush Hair ☐ Teeth

PHYSICAL THERAPY

☐ Back ☐ Neck ☐ Shoulders
☐ Arms ☐ Hands ☐ Legs ☐ Feet
☐ Speech Therapy

SPECIAL CARE

MEDICINE	DOSAGE	TIME	MEDICINE	DOSAGE	TIME
		:			:
		:			:
		:			:
		:			:
		:			:
		:			:

BLOOD PRESSURE

SYSTOLIC	DIASTOLIC	TIME
		:
		:
		:
		:
		:
		:

ACTIVITIES

ACTIVITY	LENGTH

SUPPLIES NEEDED

NOTES

LEVEL OF HAPPINESS   AM: ☐☐☐☐   PM: ☐☐☐☐
NOTES: _____
_____

LEVEL OF ENGAGEMENT   AM: ☐☐☐☐   PM: ☐☐☐☐
NOTES: _____
_____

LEVEL OF DISCOMFORT   AM: ☐☐☐☐   PM: ☐☐☐☐
NOTES: _____
_____

LEVEL OF SLEEP   AM: ☐☐☐☐   PM: ☐☐☐☐
NOTES: _____
_____

Are you noticing anything different today?
_____
_____

What is your ongoing or new goal for success in caregiving and helping your loved one to age gracefully and in a way that first their individual need and disposition?
_____
_____
_____

What were your challenges and triumphs today?
_____
_____

Do you have any questions or concerns to reach out about?
_____
_____

DATE:

TOILET / DIAPER

TIME	RESULT	
:	wet	b.m.
:	wet	b.m.
:	wet	b.m.
:	wet	b.m.
:	wet	b.m.
:	wet	b.m.
:	wet	b.m.

MEALS / FEEDINGS

TIME	AMOUNT
:	
:	
:	
:	
:	
:	
:	

PERSONAL CARE

☐ Shower   ☐ Bed Bath   ☐ Brush Hair   ☐ Teeth

PHYSICAL THERAPY

☐ Back   ☐ Neck   ☐ Shoulders
☐ Arms   ☐ Hands   ☐ Legs   ☐ Feet
☐ Speech Therapy

SPECIAL CARE

MEDICINE	DOSAGE	TIME	MEDICINE	DOSAGE	TIME
		:			:
		:			:
		:			:
		:			:
		:			:
		:			:

BLOOD PRESSURE

SYSTOLIC	DIASTOLIC	TIME
		:
		:
		:
		:
		:
		:

ACTIVITIES

ACTIVITY	LENGTH

SUPPLIES NEEDED

NOTES

LEVEL OF HAPPINESS   AM: [   ]   PM: [   ]
NOTES: _____
_____

LEVEL OF ENGAGEMENT   AM: [   ]   PM: [   ]
NOTES: _____
_____

LEVEL OF DISCOMFORT   AM: [   ]   PM: [   ]
NOTES: _____
_____

LEVEL OF SLEEP   AM: [   ]   PM: [   ]
NOTES: _____
_____

Are you noticing anything different today?
_____
_____

What is your ongoing or new goal for success in caregiving and helping your loved one to age gracefully and in a way that first their individual need and disposition?
_____
_____
_____

What were your challenges and triumphs today?
_____
_____

Do you have any questions or concerns to reach out about?
_____
_____

DATE:

TOILET / DIAPER

TIME	RESULT	
:	wet	b.m.
:	wet	b.m.
:	wet	b.m.
:	wet	b.m.
:	wet	b.m.
:	wet	b.m.
:	wet	b.m.

MEALS / FEEDINGS

TIME	AMOUNT
:	
:	
:	
:	
:	
:	
:	

PERSONAL CARE

☐ Shower ☐ Bed Bath ☐ Brush Hair ☐ Teeth

PHYSICAL THERAPY

☐ Back ☐ Neck ☐ Shoulders
☐ Arms ☐ Hands ☐ Legs ☐ Feet
☐ Speech Therapy

SPECIAL CARE

MEDICINE	DOSAGE	TIME	MEDICINE	DOSAGE	TIME
		:			:
		:			:
		:			:
		:			:
		:			:
		:			:

BLOOD PRESSURE

SYSTOLIC	DIASTOLIC	TIME
		:
		:
		:
		:
		:
		:

ACTIVITIES

ACTIVITY	LENGTH

SUPPLIES NEEDED

NOTES

LEVEL OF HAPPINESS AM: ☐☐☐☐☐ PM: ☐☐☐☐☐
NOTES: _____
_____

LEVEL OF ENGAGEMENT AM: ☐☐☐☐☐ PM: ☐☐☐☐☐
NOTES: _____
_____

LEVEL OF DISCOMFORT AM: ☐☐☐☐☐ PM: ☐☐☐☐☐
NOTES: _____
_____

LEVEL OF SLEEP AM: ☐☐☐☐☐ PM: ☐☐☐☐☐
NOTES: _____
_____

Are you noticing anything different today?
_____
_____

What is your ongoing or new goal for success in caregiving and helping your loved one to age gracefully and in a way that first their individual need and disposition?
_____
_____
_____

What were your challenges and triumphs today?
_____
_____

Do you have any questions or concerns to reach out about?
_____
_____

DATE: _____

TOILET / DIAPER

TIME	RESULT	
:	wet	b.m.
:	wet	b.m.
:	wet	b.m.
:	wet	b.m.
:	wet	b.m.
:	wet	b.m.
:	wet	b.m.

MEALS / FEEDINGS

TIME	AMOUNT
:	
:	
:	
:	
:	
:	
:	

PERSONAL CARE

☐ Shower ☐ Bed Bath ☐ Brush Hair ☐ Teeth

PHYSICAL THERAPY

☐ Back ☐ Neck ☐ Shoulders
☐ Arms ☐ Hands ☐ Legs ☐ Feet
☐ Speech Therapy

SPECIAL CARE

MEDICINE	DOSAGE	TIME	MEDICINE	DOSAGE	TIME
		:			:
		:			:
		:			:
		:			:
		:			:
		:			:

BLOOD PRESSURE

SYSTOLIC	DIASTOLIC	TIME
		:
		:
		:
		:
		:
		:

ACTIVITIES

ACTIVITY	LENGTH

SUPPLIES NEEDED

NOTES

LEVEL OF HAPPINESS AM: ☐☐☐☐☐   PM: ☐☐☐☐☐
NOTES: _____
_____

LEVEL OF ENGAGEMENT AM: ☐☐☐☐☐   PM: ☐☐☐☐☐
NOTES: _____
_____

LEVEL OF DISCOMFORT AM: ☐☐☐☐☐   PM: ☐☐☐☐☐
NOTES: _____
_____

LEVEL OF SLEEP AM: ☐☐☐☐☐   PM: ☐☐☐☐☐
NOTES: _____
_____

Are you noticing anything different today?
_____
_____

What is your ongoing or new goal for success in caregiving and helping your loved one to age gracefully and in a way that first their individual need and disposition?
_____
_____
_____

What were your challenges and triumphs today?
_____
_____

Do you have any questions or concerns to reach out about?
_____
_____

DATE:

TOILET / DIAPER

TIME	RESULT	
:	wet	b.m.
:	wet	b.m.
:	wet	b.m.
:	wet	b.m.
:	wet	b.m.
:	wet	b.m.
:	wet	b.m.

MEALS / FEEDINGS

TIME	AMOUNT
:	
:	
:	
:	
:	
:	
:	

PERSONAL CARE

☐ Shower ☐ Bed Bath ☐ Brush Hair ☐ Teeth

PHYSICAL THERAPY

☐ Back ☐ Neck ☐ Shoulders
☐ Arms ☐ Hands ☐ Legs ☐ Feet
☐ Speech Therapy

SPECIAL CARE

MEDICINE	DOSAGE	TIME	MEDICINE	DOSAGE	TIME
		:			:
		:			:
		:			:
		:			:
		:			:
		:			:

BLOOD PRESSURE

SYSTOLIC	DIASTOLIC	TIME
		:
		:
		:
		:
		:
		:

ACTIVITIES

ACTIVITY	LENGTH

SUPPLIES NEEDED

NOTES

LEVEL OF HAPPINESS AM: ☐☐☐☐ PM: ☐☐☐☐
NOTES: _____
_____

LEVEL OF ENGAGEMENT AM: ☐☐☐☐ PM: ☐☐☐☐
NOTES: _____
_____

LEVEL OF DISCOMFORT AM: ☐☐☐☐ PM: ☐☐☐☐
NOTES: _____
_____

LEVEL OF SLEEP AM: ☐☐☐☐ PM: ☐☐☐☐
NOTES: _____
_____

Are you noticing anything different today?
_____
_____

What is your ongoing or new goal for success in caregiving and helping your loved one to age gracefully and in a way that first their individual need and disposition?
_____
_____
_____

What were your challenges and triumphs today?
_____
_____

Do you have any questions or concerns to reach out about?
_____
_____

DATE:

TOILET / DIAPER

TIME	RESULT	
:	wet	b.m.
:	wet	b.m.
:	wet	b.m.
:	wet	b.m.
:	wet	b.m.
:	wet	b.m.
:	wet	b.m.

MEALS / FEEDINGS

TIME	AMOUNT
:	
:	
:	
:	
:	
:	
:	

PERSONAL CARE

☐ Shower ☐ Bed Bath ☐ Brush Hair ☐ Teeth

PHYSICAL THERAPY

☐ Back ☐ Neck ☐ Shoulders
☐ Arms ☐ Hands ☐ Legs ☐ Feet
☐ Speech Therapy

SPECIAL CARE

MEDICINE	DOSAGE	TIME	MEDICINE	DOSAGE	TIME
		:			:
		:			:
		:			:
		:			:
		:			:
		:			:

BLOOD PRESSURE

SYSTOLIC	DIASTOLIC	TIME
		:
		:
		:
		:
		:
		:

ACTIVITIES

ACTIVITY	LENGTH

SUPPLIES NEEDED

NOTES

LEVEL OF HAPPINESS   AM: ☐☐☐☐☐   PM: ☐☐☐☐☐
NOTES: _____
_____

LEVEL OF ENGAGEMENT   AM: ☐☐☐☐☐   PM: ☐☐☐☐☐
NOTES: _____
_____

LEVEL OF DISCOMFORT   AM: ☐☐☐☐☐   PM: ☐☐☐☐☐
NOTES: _____
_____

LEVEL OF SLEEP   AM: ☐☐☐☐☐   PM: ☐☐☐☐☐
NOTES: _____
_____

Are you noticing anything different today?
_____
_____

What is your ongoing or new goal for success in caregiving and helping your loved one to age gracefully and in a way that first their individual need and disposition?
_____
_____
_____

What were your challenges and triumphs today?
_____
_____

Do you have any questions or concerns to reach out about?
_____
_____

DATE:

TOILET / DIAPER

TIME	RESULT	
:	wet	b.m.
:	wet	b.m.
:	wet	b.m.
:	wet	b.m.
:	wet	b.m.
:	wet	b.m.
:	wet	b.m.

MEALS / FEEDINGS

TIME	AMOUNT
:	
:	
:	
:	
:	
:	
:	

PERSONAL CARE

☐ Shower   ☐ Bed Bath   ☐ Brush Hair   ☐ Teeth

PHYSICAL THERAPY

☐ Back   ☐ Neck   ☐ Shoulders
☐ Arms   ☐ Hands   ☐ Legs   ☐ Feet
☐ Speech Therapy

SPECIAL CARE

MEDICINE	DOSAGE	TIME	MEDICINE	DOSAGE	TIME
		:			:
		:			:
		:			:
		:			:
		:			:
		:			:

BLOOD PRESSURE

SYSTOLIC	DIASTOLIC	TIME
		:
		:
		:
		:
		:
		:

ACTIVITIES

ACTIVITY	LENGTH

SUPPLIES NEEDED

NOTES

LEVEL OF HAPPINESS   AM: ☐☐☐☐☐   PM: ☐☐☐☐☐
NOTES: _____
_____

LEVEL OF ENGAGEMENT   AM: ☐☐☐☐☐   PM: ☐☐☐☐☐
NOTES: _____
_____

LEVEL OF DISCOMFORT   AM: ☐☐☐☐☐   PM: ☐☐☐☐☐
NOTES: _____
_____

LEVEL OF SLEEP   AM: ☐☐☐☐☐   PM: ☐☐☐☐☐
NOTES: _____
_____

Are you noticing anything different today?
_____
_____

What is your ongoing or new goal for success in caregiving and helping your loved one to age gracefully and in a way that first their individual need and disposition?
_____
_____
_____

What were your challenges and triumphs today?
_____
_____

Do you have any questions or concerns to reach out about?
_____
_____

DATE:

TOILET / DIAPER

TIME	RESULT	
:	wet	b.m.
:	wet	b.m.
:	wet	b.m.
:	wet	b.m.
:	wet	b.m.
:	wet	b.m.
:	wet	b.m.

MEALS / FEEDINGS

TIME	AMOUNT
:	
:	
:	
:	
:	
:	
:	

PERSONAL CARE

☐ Shower ☐ Bed Bath ☐ Brush Hair ☐ Teeth

PHYSICAL THERAPY

☐ Back   ☐ Neck   ☐ Shoulders
☐ Arms   ☐ Hands   ☐ Legs   ☐ Feet
☐ Speech Therapy

SPECIAL CARE

MEDICINE	DOSAGE	TIME	MEDICINE	DOSAGE	TIME
		:			:
		:			:
		:			:
		:			:
		:			:
		:			:

BLOOD PRESSURE

SYSTOLIC	DIASTOLIC	TIME
		:
		:
		:
		:
		:
		:

ACTIVITIES

ACTIVITY	LENGTH

SUPPLIES NEEDED

NOTES

LEVEL OF HAPPINESS   AM: ☐☐☐☐   PM: ☐☐☐☐
NOTES: _____
_____

LEVEL OF ENGAGEMENT   AM: ☐☐☐☐   PM: ☐☐☐☐
NOTES: _____
_____

LEVEL OF DISCOMFORT   AM: ☐☐☐☐   PM: ☐☐☐☐
NOTES: _____
_____

LEVEL OF SLEEP   AM: ☐☐☐☐   PM: ☐☐☐☐
NOTES: _____
_____

Are you noticing anything different today?
_____
_____

What is your ongoing or new goal for success in caregiving and helping your loved one to age gracefully and in a way that first their individual need and disposition?
_____
_____
_____

What were your challenges and triumphs today?
_____
_____

Do you have any questions or concerns to reach out about?
_____
_____

DATE: _____

TOILET / DIAPER

TIME	RESULT	
:	wet	b.m.
:	wet	b.m.
:	wet	b.m.
:	wet	b.m.
:	wet	b.m.
:	wet	b.m.
:	wet	b.m.

MEALS / FEEDINGS

TIME	AMOUNT
:	
:	
:	
:	
:	
:	
:	

PERSONAL CARE

☐ Shower ☐ Bed Bath ☐ Brush Hair ☐ Teeth

PHYSICAL THERAPY

☐ Back ☐ Neck ☐ Shoulders
☐ Arms ☐ Hands ☐ Legs ☐ Feet
☐ Speech Therapy

SPECIAL CARE

MEDICINE	DOSAGE	TIME	MEDICINE	DOSAGE	TIME
		:			:
		:			:
		:			:
		:			:
		:			:
		:			:

BLOOD PRESSURE

SYSTOLIC	DIASTOLIC	TIME
		:
		:
		:
		:
		:
		:

ACTIVITIES

ACTIVITY	LENGTH

SUPPLIES NEEDED

NOTES

LEVEL OF HAPPINESS AM: ☐☐☐☐ PM: ☐☐☐☐
NOTES: _____
_____

LEVEL OF ENGAGEMENT AM: ☐☐☐☐ PM: ☐☐☐☐
NOTES: _____
_____

LEVEL OF DISCOMFORT AM: ☐☐☐☐ PM: ☐☐☐☐
NOTES: _____
_____

LEVEL OF SLEEP AM: ☐☐☐☐ PM: ☐☐☐☐
NOTES: _____
_____

Are you noticing anything different today?
_____
_____

What is your ongoing or new goal for success in caregiving and helping your loved one to age gracefully and in a way that first their individual need and disposition?
_____
_____
_____

What were your challenges and triumphs today?
_____
_____

Do you have any questions or concerns to reach out about?
_____
_____

DATE:

TOILET / DIAPER

TIME	RESULT	
:	wet	b.m.
:	wet	b.m.
:	wet	b.m.
:	wet	b.m.
:	wet	b.m.
:	wet	b.m.
:	wet	b.m.

MEALS / FEEDINGS

TIME	AMOUNT
:	
:	
:	
:	
:	
:	
:	

PERSONAL CARE

☐ Shower ☐ Bed Bath ☐ Brush Hair ☐ Teeth

PHYSICAL THERAPY

☐ Back ☐ Neck ☐ Shoulders
☐ Arms ☐ Hands ☐ Legs ☐ Feet
☐ Speech Therapy

SPECIAL CARE

MEDICINE	DOSAGE	TIME	MEDICINE	DOSAGE	TIME
		:			:
		:			:
		:			:
		:			:
		:			:
		:			:

BLOOD PRESSURE

SYSTOLIC	DIASTOLIC	TIME
		:
		:
		:
		:
		:
		:

ACTIVITIES

ACTIVITY	LENGTH

SUPPLIES NEEDED

NOTES

LEVEL OF HAPPINESS   AM: ☐☐☐☐☐   PM: ☐☐☐☐☐
NOTES: _____
_____

LEVEL OF ENGAGEMENT   AM: ☐☐☐☐☐   PM: ☐☐☐☐☐
NOTES: _____
_____

LEVEL OF DISCOMFORT   AM: ☐☐☐☐☐   PM: ☐☐☐☐☐
NOTES: _____
_____

LEVEL OF SLEEP   AM: ☐☐☐☐☐   PM: ☐☐☐☐☐
NOTES: _____
_____

Are you noticing anything different today?
_____
_____

What is your ongoing or new goal for success in caregiving and helping your loved one to age gracefully and in a way that first their individual need and disposition?
_____
_____
_____

What were your challenges and triumphs today?
_____
_____

Do you have any questions or concerns to reach out about?
_____
_____

DATE:

TOILET / DIAPER

TIME	RESULT	
:	wet	b.m.
:	wet	b.m.
:	wet	b.m.
:	wet	b.m.
:	wet	b.m.
:	wet	b.m.
:	wet	b.m.

MEALS / FEEDINGS

TIME	AMOUNT
:	
:	
:	
:	
:	
:	
:	

PERSONAL CARE

☐ Shower ☐ Bed Bath ☐ Brush Hair ☐ Teeth

PHYSICAL THERAPY

☐ Back ☐ Neck ☐ Shoulders
☐ Arms ☐ Hands ☐ Legs ☐ Feet
☐ Speech Therapy

SPECIAL CARE

MEDICINE	DOSAGE	TIME	MEDICINE	DOSAGE	TIME
		:			:
		:			:
		:			:
		:			:
		:			:
		:			:

BLOOD PRESSURE

SYSTOLIC	DIASTOLIC	TIME
		:
		:
		:
		:
		:
		:

ACTIVITIES

ACTIVITY	LENGTH

SUPPLIES NEEDED

NOTES

LEVEL OF HAPPINESS　　AM: ☐☐☐☐☐　　PM: ☐☐☐☐☐
NOTES: _____
_____

LEVEL OF ENGAGEMENT　AM: ☐☐☐☐☐　　PM: ☐☐☐☐☐
NOTES: _____
_____

LEVEL OF DISCOMFORT　AM: ☐☐☐☐☐　　PM: ☐☐☐☐☐
NOTES: _____
_____

LEVEL OF SLEEP　　　　AM: ☐☐☐☐☐　　PM: ☐☐☐☐☐
NOTES: _____
_____

Are you noticing anything different today?
_____
_____

What is your ongoing or new goal for success in caregiving and helping your loved one to age gracefully and in a way that first their individual need and disposition?
_____
_____
_____

What were your challenges and triumphs today?
_____
_____

Do you have any questions or concerns to reach out about?
_____
_____

DATE:

TOILET / DIAPER

TIME	RESULT	
:	wet	b.m.
:	wet	b.m.
:	wet	b.m.
:	wet	b.m.
:	wet	b.m.
:	wet	b.m.
:	wet	b.m.

MEALS / FEEDINGS

TIME	AMOUNT
:	
:	
:	
:	
:	
:	
:	

PERSONAL CARE

☐ Shower   ☐ Bed Bath   ☐ Brush Hair   ☐ Teeth

PHYSICAL THERAPY

☐ Back   ☐ Neck   ☐ Shoulders
☐ Arms   ☐ Hands   ☐ Legs   ☐ Feet
☐ Speech Therapy

SPECIAL CARE

MEDICINE	DOSAGE	TIME	MEDICINE	DOSAGE	TIME
		:			:
		:			:
		:			:
		:			:
		:			:
		:			:

BLOOD PRESSURE

SYSTOLIC	DIASTOLIC	TIME
		:
		:
		:
		:
		:
		:

ACTIVITIES

ACTIVITY	LENGTH

SUPPLIES NEEDED

NOTES

LEVEL OF HAPPINESS   AM: ☐☐☐☐☐   PM: ☐☐☐☐☐
NOTES: _____
_____

LEVEL OF ENGAGEMENT   AM: ☐☐☐☐☐   PM: ☐☐☐☐☐
NOTES: _____
_____

LEVEL OF DISCOMFORT   AM: ☐☐☐☐☐   PM: ☐☐☐☐☐
NOTES: _____
_____

LEVEL OF SLEEP   AM: ☐☐☐☐☐   PM: ☐☐☐☐☐
NOTES: _____
_____

Are you noticing anything different today?
_____
_____

What is your ongoing or new goal for success in caregiving and helping your loved one to age gracefully and in a way that first their individual need and disposition?
_____
_____
_____

What were your challenges and triumphs today?
_____
_____

Do you have any questions or concerns to reach out about?
_____
_____

DATE:

TOILET / DIAPER

TIME	RESULT	
:	wet	b.m.
:	wet	b.m.
:	wet	b.m.
:	wet	b.m.
:	wet	b.m.
:	wet	b.m.
:	wet	b.m.

MEALS / FEEDINGS

TIME	AMOUNT
:	
:	
:	
:	
:	
:	
:	

PERSONAL CARE

☐ Shower ☐ Bed Bath ☐ Brush Hair ☐ Teeth

PHYSICAL THERAPY

☐ Back ☐ Neck ☐ Shoulders
☐ Arms ☐ Hands ☐ Legs ☐ Feet
☐ Speech Therapy

SPECIAL CARE

MEDICINE	DOSAGE	TIME	MEDICINE	DOSAGE	TIME
		:			:
		:			:
		:			:
		:			:
		:			:
		:			:

BLOOD PRESSURE

SYSTOLIC	DIASTOLIC	TIME
		:
		:
		:
		:
		:
		:

ACTIVITIES

ACTIVITY	LENGTH

SUPPLIES NEEDED

NOTES

LEVEL OF HAPPINESS AM: ▢▢▢▢▢   PM: ▢▢▢▢▢
NOTES: _____
_____

LEVEL OF ENGAGEMENT AM: ▢▢▢▢▢   PM: ▢▢▢▢▢
NOTES: _____
_____

LEVEL OF DISCOMFORT AM: ▢▢▢▢▢   PM: ▢▢▢▢▢
NOTES: _____
_____

LEVEL OF SLEEP AM: ▢▢▢▢▢   PM: ▢▢▢▢▢
NOTES: _____
_____

Are you noticing anything different today?
_____
_____

What is your ongoing or new goal for success in caregiving and helping your loved one to age gracefully and in a way that first their individual need and disposition?
_____
_____
_____

What were your challenges and triumphs today?
_____
_____

Do you have any questions or concerns to reach out about?
_____
_____

DATE:

TOILET / DIAPER

TIME	RESULT	
:	wet	b.m.
:	wet	b.m.
:	wet	b.m.
:	wet	b.m.
:	wet	b.m.
:	wet	b.m.
:	wet	b.m.

MEALS / FEEDINGS

TIME	AMOUNT
:	
:	
:	
:	
:	
:	
:	

PERSONAL CARE

☐ Shower ☐ Bed Bath ☐ Brush Hair ☐ Teeth

PHYSICAL THERAPY

☐ Back ☐ Neck ☐ Shoulders
☐ Arms ☐ Hands ☐ Legs ☐ Feet
☐ Speech Therapy

SPECIAL CARE

MEDICINE	DOSAGE	TIME	MEDICINE	DOSAGE	TIME
		:			:
		:			:
		:			:
		:			:
		:			:
		:			:

BLOOD PRESSURE

SYSTOLIC	DIASTOLIC	TIME
		:
		:
		:
		:
		:
		:

ACTIVITIES

ACTIVITY	LENGTH

SUPPLIES NEEDED

NOTES

LEVEL OF HAPPINESS   AM: ☐☐☐☐☐   PM: ☐☐☐☐☐
NOTES: _____
_____

LEVEL OF ENGAGEMENT   AM: ☐☐☐☐☐   PM: ☐☐☐☐☐
NOTES: _____
_____

LEVEL OF DISCOMFORT   AM: ☐☐☐☐☐   PM: ☐☐☐☐☐
NOTES: _____
_____

LEVEL OF SLEEP   AM: ☐☐☐☐☐   PM: ☐☐☐☐☐
NOTES: _____
_____

Are you noticing anything different today?
_____
_____

What is your ongoing or new goal for success in caregiving and helping your loved one to age gracefully and in a way that first their individual need and disposition?
_____
_____
_____

What were your challenges and triumphs today?
_____
_____

Do you have any questions or concerns to reach out about?
_____
_____

DATE:

TOILET / DIAPER

TIME	RESULT	
:	wet	b.m.
:	wet	b.m.
:	wet	b.m.
:	wet	b.m.
:	wet	b.m.
:	wet	b.m.
:	wet	b.m.

MEALS / FEEDINGS

TIME	AMOUNT
:	
:	
:	
:	
:	
:	
:	

PERSONAL CARE

☐ Shower ☐ Bed Bath ☐ Brush Hair ☐ Teeth

PHYSICAL THERAPY

☐ Back ☐ Neck ☐ Shoulders
☐ Arms ☐ Hands ☐ Legs ☐ Feet
☐ Speech Therapy

SPECIAL CARE

MEDICINE	DOSAGE	TIME	MEDICINE	DOSAGE	TIME
		:			:
		:			:
		:			:
		:			:
		:			:
		:			:

BLOOD PRESSURE

SYSTOLIC	DIASTOLIC	TIME
		:
		:
		:
		:
		:
		:

ACTIVITIES

ACTIVITY	LENGTH

SUPPLIES NEEDED

NOTES

LEVEL OF HAPPINESS   AM: ☐☐☐☐☐   PM: ☐☐☐☐☐
NOTES: _____
_____

LEVEL OF ENGAGEMENT   AM: ☐☐☐☐☐   PM: ☐☐☐☐☐
NOTES: _____
_____

LEVEL OF DISCOMFORT   AM: ☐☐☐☐☐   PM: ☐☐☐☐☐
NOTES: _____
_____

LEVEL OF SLEEP   AM: ☐☐☐☐☐   PM: ☐☐☐☐☐
NOTES: _____
_____

Are you noticing anything different today?
_____
_____

What is your ongoing or new goal for success in caregiving and helping your loved one to age gracefully and in a way that first their individual need and disposition?
_____
_____
_____

What were your challenges and triumphs today?
_____
_____

Do you have any questions or concerns to reach out about?
_____
_____

DATE:

TOILET / DIAPER

TIME	RESULT	
:	wet	b.m.
:	wet	b.m.
:	wet	b.m.
:	wet	b.m.
:	wet	b.m.
:	wet	b.m.
:	wet	b.m.

MEALS / FEEDINGS

TIME	AMOUNT
:	
:	
:	
:	
:	
:	
:	

PERSONAL CARE

☐ Shower ☐ Bed Bath ☐ Brush Hair ☐ Teeth

PHYSICAL THERAPY

☐ Back ☐ Neck ☐ Shoulders
☐ Arms ☐ Hands ☐ Legs ☐ Feet
☐ Speech Therapy

SPECIAL CARE

MEDICINE	DOSAGE	TIME	MEDICINE	DOSAGE	TIME
		:			:
		:			:
		:			:
		:			:
		:			:
		:			:

BLOOD PRESSURE

SYSTOLIC	DIASTOLIC	TIME
		:
		:
		:
		:
		:
		:

ACTIVITIES

ACTIVITY	LENGTH

SUPPLIES NEEDED

NOTES

LEVEL OF HAPPINESS   AM: ☐☐☐☐☐   PM: ☐☐☐☐☐
NOTES: _____
_____

LEVEL OF ENGAGEMENT   AM: ☐☐☐☐☐   PM: ☐☐☐☐☐
NOTES: _____
_____

LEVEL OF DISCOMFORT   AM: ☐☐☐☐☐   PM: ☐☐☐☐☐
NOTES: _____
_____

LEVEL OF SLEEP   AM: ☐☐☐☐☐   PM: ☐☐☐☐☐
NOTES: _____
_____

Are you noticing anything different today?
_____
_____

What is your ongoing or new goal for success in caregiving and helping your loved one to age gracefully and in a way that first their individual need and disposition?
_____
_____
_____

What were your challenges and triumphs today?
_____
_____

Do you have any questions or concerns to reach out about?
_____
_____

DATE:

TOILET / DIAPER

TIME	RESULT	
:	wet	b.m.
:	wet	b.m.
:	wet	b.m.
:	wet	b.m.
:	wet	b.m.
:	wet	b.m.
:	wet	b.m.

MEALS / FEEDINGS

TIME	AMOUNT
:	
:	
:	
:	
:	
:	
:	

PERSONAL CARE

☐ Shower ☐ Bed Bath ☐ Brush Hair ☐ Teeth

PHYSICAL THERAPY

☐ Back   ☐ Neck   ☐ Shoulders

☐ Arms   ☐ Hands   ☐ Legs   ☐ Feet

☐ Speech Therapy

SPECIAL CARE

MEDICINE	DOSAGE	TIME	MEDICINE	DOSAGE	TIME
		:			:
		:			:
		:			:
		:			:
		:			:
		:			:

BLOOD PRESSURE

SYSTOLIC	DIASTOLIC	TIME
		:
		:
		:
		:
		:
		:

ACTIVITIES

ACTIVITY	LENGTH

SUPPLIES NEEDED

NOTES

LEVEL OF HAPPINESS AM: ☐☐☐☐☐ PM: ☐☐☐☐☐
NOTES: _____
_____

LEVEL OF ENGAGEMENT AM: ☐☐☐☐☐ PM: ☐☐☐☐☐
NOTES: _____
_____

LEVEL OF DISCOMFORT AM: ☐☐☐☐☐ PM: ☐☐☐☐☐
NOTES: _____
_____

LEVEL OF SLEEP AM: ☐☐☐☐☐ PM: ☐☐☐☐☐
NOTES: _____
_____

Are you noticing anything different today?
_____
_____

What is your ongoing or new goal for success in caregiving and helping your loved one to age gracefully and in a way that first their individual need and disposition?
_____
_____
_____

What were your challenges and triumphs today?
_____
_____

Do you have any questions or concerns to reach out about?
_____
_____

TELEPHONE CONTACT LIST

FIRST NAME	LAST NAME	WORK PHONE	CELL PHONE	HOME PHONE

TELEPHONE CONTACT LIST

FIRST NAME	LAST NAME	WORK PHONE	CELL PHONE	HOME PHONE

www.ingramcontent.com/pod-product-compliance
Lightning Source LLC
Chambersburg PA
CBHW081620100526
44590CB00021B/3530